Regional Anesthesia

Techniques and Clinical Applications

REGIONAL ANESTHESIA

Techniques and Clinical Applications

Harold Carron, M.D.
Professor of Anesthesiology
Consultant, Pain Management Center

Gregg A. Korbon, M.D.
Assistant Professor of Anesthesiology
Attending Physician, Pain Management Center

John C. Rowlingson, M.D.
Associate Professor of Anesthesiology
Director, Pain Management Center

Department of Anesthesiology
University of Virginia Medical Center
Charlottesville, Virginia

GRUNE & STRATTON, INC.
Harcourt Brace Jovanovich, Publishers
Orlando   New York   San Diego   Boston   London
San Francisco   Tokyo   Sydney   Toronto

Library of Congress Cataloging in Publication Data

Carron, Harold, 1916–
  Regional anesthesia.

  Bibliography: p. 185.
  Includes index.
  1. Conduction anesthesia. I. Korbon, Gregg A.
II. Rowlingson, John C. III. Title. [DNLM: 1. Anes-
thesia, Conduction—methods. WO 300 C319r]
RD84.C37 1984   617′.964   84-12806
ISBN 0-8089-1654-8

Grune & Stratton, Inc.
Orlando, Florida 32887

Distributed in the United Kingdom by
Grune & Stratton, Ltd.
24/28 Oval Road, London NW 1

Library of Congress Catalog Number 84-12806
International Standard Book Number 0-8089-1654-8

Printed in the United States of America
85 86 87 10 9 8 7 6 5 4 3 2

This book is dedicated to all physicians, particularly neophyte anesthesiology residents who are learning new techniques to provide better care for their patients.

Contents

Acknowledgments

The authors are pleased to acknowledge the introductory chapter on pharmacology and toxicity of local anesthetics by Cosmo A. DiFazio, M.D., Ph.D., and the assistance of Joanne Stanley for both compilation of material and editing of manuscripts.

We further wish to acknowledge the writings and research of the pioneers in anesthesia who have laid the groundwork for our own knowledge and teaching of regional anesthesia. Some of the procedures described have been previously published by other authors, but, in general, techniques have been modified, simplified, or refined to conform to safe practice and success in performance.

We are greatly indebted to Keith W. Shahan for the photography and to Linda B. Hamme for the superb drawings, both of which were essential for this text. Recognition is made of the assistance of various members of the Department of Anesthesiology of the University of Virginia Medical Center in providing facilities and in acting as models for demonstrations of nerve blocking techniques.

The cooperation of Grune & Stratton is acknowledged for encouraging us to expand a chapter entitled "Common Nerve Blocks in Anesthetic Practice" (*Seminars in Anesthesia*, Vol. II, No. 1, March 1983) to a more comprehensive volume.

Preface

Regional anesthesia has many advantages over general anesthetic techniques when the procedure is tailored to the particular patient and the proposed surgery. Recent studies have shown that regional techniques may also be valuable in modulating stress responses of surgery, especially in the postoperative period.

The purpose of this text is to provide the anesthesiologist, surgeon, and medical practitioner with useful and clearly defined guidelines on the pertinent anatomical considerations, surface landmarks, and techniques for performing regional anesthetic procedures. Photographs depict superficial anatomical landmarks. Cutaway drawings illustrate the relationship of the surface landmarks to the nerves to be blocked. In some instances, deep landmarks will be drawn to indicate structures neither observable nor palpable. Other drawings depict the area of anesthesia produced with each block. While the format may appear somewhat "cookbook" in style, it is the authors' opinion that for successful regional anesthesia it is essential that a reproducible routine be established.

This book is organized in sections by type of block. In each chapter, potential complications of a procedure are discussed following the sectins on anatomy, landmarks, and technique of that block. Section V provides suggestions for improving accuracy and quality of blocks. Section VI discusses complications in general, with recommendations on their avoidance and management. Not all theoretically possible nerve blocks are included in this treatise. Those blocks that are rarely performed have been omitted; in the hands of the neophyte, their success rates may be discouraging.

Indications for each block described are assumed to have been determined after discussion with the surgeon as to the extent of the surgical procedure, and with the patient as to the advantages, technique, and complications of the block. A pre-block physical examination, with particular reference to the site of proposed needle insertion, is essential to determine anatomical variations, the presence of skin lesions, neurological deficits, or physical limitations that may prevent successful performance of the block. For each nerve block described, it should be determined that no contraindication exists to needle-invasive procedures (tumor, infection, coagulopathy), and premedication should be used judiciously with the purpose of allaying apprehension rather than producing analgesia or amnesia. Absorption of local anesthetic into the systemic circulation often provides additional analgesia and sedation in and of itself.

It is assumed that all blocks will be performed under aseptic technique, and that proper limitation of drug dosages as outlined in this book will be observed. Both the anesthesiologist and surgeon must be prepared for the delay in the block "setting up." The onset of neural blockade should be checked after five minutes for level of analgesia using cold rather than needle prick. The loss of cold sensation precedes loss of pinprick sensation by several minutes and therefore provides an earlier indication of adequacy and extent of block. This allows supplementation of the block as necessary, thereby assuring a higher degree of success.

Equipment must be on hand to provide supplementary general anesthesia or further regional procedures as needed. Immediate availability of drugs and equipment is essential for the treatment of untoward reactions and systemic toxicity. Minimal requirements are an oxygen source with bag and mask for ventilation, endotracheal intubation equipment, intravenous solutions, and an in-syringe supply of sodium pentobarbital, diazepam, succinylcholine, and vasopressors.

Careful attention to detail and accurate needle placement as described in this text will result in dense blocks utilizing minimal drug concentrations and volumes. Regional anesthesia confidently and properly applied to an informed surgical patient will result in less physiologic derangement, greater patient comfort, and shortened convalescence.

List of Illustrations

Regional Anesthesia

Techniques and Clinical Applications

Introduction

Pharmacology of Local Anesthetics and Choice of Agent

Cosmo A. DiFazio, M.D., Ph.D.

GENERAL CHEMISTRY

Local anesthetics are commonly used to reversibly inhibit nerve conduction in all types of neurons. Clinically, these drugs essentially fall into two categories: *ester*-linked tertiary amines, or *amide*-linked tertiary amines. The structures and properties of representative drugs are shown in Figure I-1. The features common to all these drugs are listed below:

1. An aromatic moiety which is lipophilic. This allows the molecule to pass through the lipid-containing cell membrane to the site of action.
2. An amino group with three organic groups attached (tertiary amine). The amino group will become charged (ionized) with the addition of a hydrogen ion. The pKa values (pKa is the pH where 50% of the drug is ionized) all fall in the narrow range from 7.6–8.9. In body fluids at physiologic pH, the charged drug

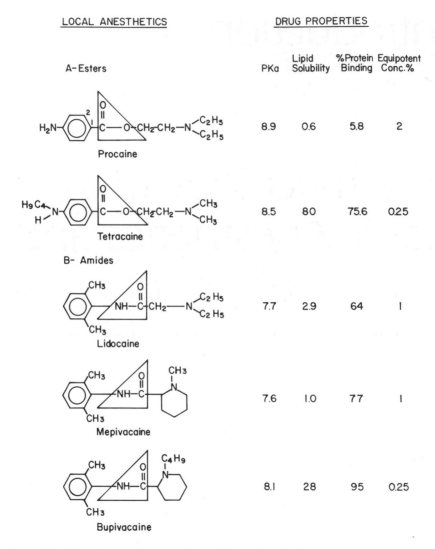

	PKa	Lipid Solubility	%Protein Binding	Equipotent Conc.%
A–Esters				
Procaine	8.9	0.6	5.8	2
Tetracaine	8.5	80	75.6	0.25
B– Amides				
Lidocaine	7.7	2.9	64	1
Mepivacaine	7.6	1.0	77	1
Bupivacaine	8.1	28	95	0.25

Figure I-1. Structure and properties of local anesthetics.

predominates and it is the active form providing neural blockade at the site of action.
3. An ester or amide link is present between the lipophilic group
and the amino group. The type of link determines the site of
metabolic inactivation of the drug. The ester-linked drugs are
inactivated in plasma while the amide-linked drugs must get to
the liver before inactivation takes place.

LOCAL ANESTHETIC ACTION ON NERVES

Electrical signals in excitable tissues are the result of propagated ionic currents, which are created by transient alterations in the gradient for several ionic species. The ionic concentration of sodium (Na^+) is large extracellularly and low intracellularly while that of potassium (K^+) is large intracellularly and low extracellularly. The resting potential of about -90 mV is largely the result of the K^+ conductance which at rest is very much greater than Na^+ conductance. The ionic gradient of K^+ and Na^+ across the cell membrane is maintained by an ion-translocating $Na^+ - K^+$ ATPase pump mechanism.

In studies including Hodgkin and Huxley voltage clamp experiments, the initial upswing in an action potential in nerve conduction was found to be caused by an increase in the sodium ion permeability of the nerve membrane with a resultant inward movement of sodium ions in specific ion channels.[1,2] A stimulus leading to an action potential causes the voltage-dependent sodium channel to open, which increases Na^+ conductance with the sodium ions moving intracellularly with depolarization. Several investigators have postulated that the action potential causes a conformational change in the nerve membrane lipoprotein.[3,4] This conformational change results in the opening of a channel within the lipoprotein structure which, because of size and change, is ion-specific. The above-threshold spike produced ends with closure of the sodium channel and the intrinsic inactivation of Na^+ conductance. Depolarization spreads to adjacent membrane areas which reach threshold voltage and propagate the action potential. Potassium ion outflow commences after completion of the sodium ion movement and both ions are subsequently restored to initial intra- and extra-cellular concentrations by the sodium–potassium ATPase pump mechanism after completion of the action potential.

The local anesthetics prevent formation of the action potential by blocking the sodium channel. The anesthesia which results has been referred to as membrane stabilization; that is, the resting membrane potential is unaffected by nerve stimulation. The inhibition of the ionic movement in the sodium channel by local anesthetics could result from one of several mechanisms which can alter access to or movement within the sodium channel:

1. Biotoxins such as tetrodotoxin and saxitoxin produce a local anesthetic effect when applied in nanomolar concentrations to the external surface of the nerve membrane. These local anesthetics could become attached to the *mouth* of the sodium channel on the extracellular surface of the channel and prevent the influx of sodium ions that is associated with an action potential

from this site. This is felt to be their site of action.

2. The ester- and amide-type local anesthetics most likely act by binding of the local anesthetic *within* the sodium channel with the local anesthetic entering the channel from the axoplasmic (intracellular) side of the nerve membrane. Considerable evidence has been amassed to indicate that the ester and amide local anesthetics penetrate the cell membrane in a lipid-soluble uncharged form and reequilibrate into both charged cationic and free base (uncharged form) in accordance with their pKa and the fluid pH in the axoplasm of the nerve. The charged local anesthetic then enters the sodium channel from the intracellular side of the channel, binds to an anionic site within the channel and physically or ionically blocks sodium movement within the channel. This would be the hydrophilic pathway of the Hille[5] unitary theory for the site of action of local anesthetics.

3. Blockade of the sodium channel by membrane expansion has been proposed as the mechanism of action of the local anesthetics which are not tertiary amines, such as benzocaine. In this hypothesis, these local anesthetics dissolve in the nerve membrane in their lipophilic free base form and cause disorder (or fluidization) of the cell membrane, which in turn causes an increased external pressure on the sodium channel with resultant channel distortion and loss of channel function. These uncharged local anesthetics could also move after being dissolved in the lipid portion of the nerve membrane and diffuse directly to the receptor site in the sodium channel. This would be the hydrophobic pathway of the Hille unitary theory.

The lipid solubility of the local anesthetic is the primary determinant of the potency of the local anesthetic. It will also determine the amount dissolved in the cell membrane. The protein binding of the local anesthetic relates well with the duration of action of the drug.

The duration of action of local anesthetics is also proportional to the time that the drug remains in contact with the nerve tissues. The addition of epinephrine 1:200,000 (5 µg/ml) will decrease local tissue blood flow and retard drug absorption from the site of action. In general, this will increase the duration of local anesthetic blockade of the nerve and also result in 25% lower blood levels of the local anesthetic. These effects of the combination of epinephrine with local anesthetics occur with all local anesthetics when used for peripheral nerve blocks; i.e., infiltration and nerve conduction blocks. When the local anesthetics are used for epidural anesthesia, epinephrine will reduce absorption and prolong the block produced by the local anesthetics for all but bupivacaine and etidocaine which, because of their high lipid solubility, have delayed vascular uptake. Caution must be exercised, however, in the use of epinephrine in hypertensive patients. The suggested maximal doses for the commonly used local anesthetics are shown in Table I-1.

These doses should result in blood concentrations that are one-half that which produces seizures when used for anesthesia in areas as vascular as the epidural space.

DRUG BIOTRANSFORMATION

Ester-linked local anesthetics are hydrolyzed in plasma by plasma cholinesterase (more commonly referred to as plasma pseudocholinesterase). The enzyme has no known function in the body, but is known to hydrolyze choline esters including succinylcholine and ester-linked local anesthetics.[6] The rate of hydrolysis of the ester local anesthetics will depend on the substitution on the aromatic ring of the structure. The half-life in plasma will vary from less than 1 minute for 2-chloroprocaine to about 8 minutes for tetracaine. In the presence of an atypical pseudocholinesterase, hydrolysis of the ester-linked local anesthetics is markedly decreased. The result is that the half-life of the drug in plasma is markedly prolonged and the potential for systemic toxicity with repeat injections becomes increasingly greater.

The amide-linked local anesthetics are transported to the liver by the circulation. Biotransformation occurs in the liver. The major factors controlling clearance of the amide-linked local anesthetics by the liver include *hepatic blood flow* (amount delivered to the liver) and *drug extraction* by the liver. Decreased hepatic blood flow can be caused by the concomitant administration of general anesthetics, propranolol, and norepinephrine.[7,8,9] Drug extraction by the liver also will be decreased

Table I-1
Suggested Maximal Doses of Commonly Used Anesthetics

	Plain	With Epinephrine
	(mg/kg)	(mg/kg)
2-Chloroprocaine	20	25
Procaine	14	18
Lidocaine	7	9
Mepivacaine	7	9
Bupivacaine	2	3
Tetracaine	1.5	2

when liver function is decreased, such as when congestive heart failure or cirrhosis is present or when body temperature is decreased.[10] In addition, local anesthetic extraction by the liver may also be decreased by the concomitant administration of cimetidine. Decreases in hepatic blood flow or hepatic extraction of local anesthetic will prolong the half-life of amide-linked local anesthetics. The half-life of all amide local anesthetics is much longer than the ester-linked anesthetics and varies from 1.5 to 2.7 hours depending on which amide local anesthetic is used.

DRUG SELECTION

The selection of the local anesthetic and the concentration to use will depend on several factors such as the site of surgery, the duration of the procedure, and the physical status of the patient. In general, higher concentrations of local anesthetics are associated with a more rapid onset and a higher density of block and a longer duration of sensory blockade. A greater incidence of motor blockade of the nerves also occurs with higher concentrations. In general, central neural blocks such as spinal or epidural blocks will have a shorter duration of action than that produced in major peripheral blocks such as brachial plexus blocks when similar drug concentrations are used.

In summary, local anesthetics are extremely useful drugs. For anesthesiologists, they are primarily used to produce reversible neural blockade by their direct application to nerves. This effect is produced by a membrane-stabilizing effect on the nerve membrane through altering the sodium channel. The time to onset and duration of action of the local anesthetic is concentration-dependent and can be altered by the addition of epinephrine to the local anesthetic solution. Toxicity of the local anesthetics in the brain and cardiovascular system is blood-concentration-dependent which in turn is dose-dependent. The local anesthetics have a considerable margin of safety between effective and toxic doses. ■

REFERENCES

1. Hodgkin AL, Huxley AF: A quantitative description of membrane current and its application to conduction and excitation in nerve. J Physiol (Lond) 117:500, 1952
2. Narahasi T, Yamanda M, Frazier DT: Cationic forms of local anesthetics block action potentials from inside the nerve membrane. Nature, 223:748, 1969

3. Metcalfe JC, Burgen ASV: Relaxation of anesthetics in the presence of cyto-membranes. Nature, 220:587, 1968

4. Shanes AM: Electrochemical aspects of physiological and pharmacological action in excitable cells. II. The action potential and excitation. Pharmacol Rev 10:165, 1958

5. Hille B: Local anesthetics: Hydrophilic and hydrophobic pathways for the drug-recepter action. J Gen Physiol 69:497, 1977

6. Foldes FF, Davidson FM, Duncalf D, Kuwabara S: The intravenous toxicity of local anesthetics in man. Clin Pharmacol Ther 6:328, 1965

7. Munson ES, Tucker WK, Ausinsch B, Malagodi H: Etidocaine, bupivacaine and lidocaine seizure thresholds in monkeys. Anesthesiology 42:471, 1975

8. Burney RG, DiFazio CA: Hepatic clearance of lidocaine during N_2O anesthesia in dogs. Anesth Analg 55:322, 1976

9. Benowitz N, Forsyth RP, Melmon KL, Rowland M: Lidocaine disposition kinetics in monkeys and man. II. Effect of hemorrhage and sympathomimetic drug administration. Clin Pharmacol Ther 16:99, 1974

10. Branch RA, Shand DG, Wilkinson GR, Nies AS: The reduction of lidocaine clearance by dl-propranolol: An example of hemodynamic drug interaction. J Pharmacol Exp Ther 184:515, 1973

Section 1

Plexus Blocks

1

Cervical Plexus Blocks

B lock of the nerves arising from the cervical plexus produces anesthesia for most surgical procedures on the neck. The superficial
cervical block is used for superficial procedures and the deep
cervical block where invasion of deeper structures is contemplated.

Anatomy

The cervical nerves leave the intervertebral foramina behind the
vertebral artery and lie in the sulci of the transverse processes of C2, 3,
and 4. The anterior processes of these nerves join to form the cervical
plexus, which passes between the anterior and medial scalene muscles
to curve around the posterior border of the sternocleidomastoid muscle
which lies superficial to the transverse processes at that point. On
exiting the posterior border of the sternocleidomastoid muscle, the
cervical plexus divides to provide innervation to the skin and superficial
tissues from the lower border of the mandible to just below the clavicle,
to the midline anteriorly, and posteriorly to involve the posterior cervical
and occipital regions.

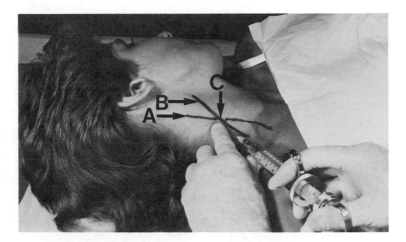

Figure 1-1. Superficial cervical plexus block: **A** represents the posterior border of the sternocleidomastoid muscle, **B** the external jugular vein, and **C** the intersection of **A** and **B,** the point of entry of the needle. Injection is carried out in a fanwise manner just beneath the posterior border of the muscle.

SUPERFICIAL CERVICAL PLEXUS BLOCK

Landmarks

With the patient in the supine position and the head slightly elevated on a folded sheet or towel, the head is then extended and rotated to the side opposite to be blocked to outline the sternocleidomastoid muscle. The point of needle entry (Fig. 1-1) lies where the external jugular vein crosses the posterior border of the muscle.

Technique

The needle is inserted at the above point and 15 ml of local anesthetic is injected in a fan-wise manner under the external jugular vein and behind the posterior border of the sternocleidomastoid muscle (Fig. 1-2). The area of anesthesia produced is shown in Figure 1-3.

DEEP CERVICAL PLEXUS BLOCK

Landmarks

The patient is positioned similarly as for the superficial plexus block with the head extended and rotated to the side away from that to be blocked. The lower tip of the mastoid process which overlies the first

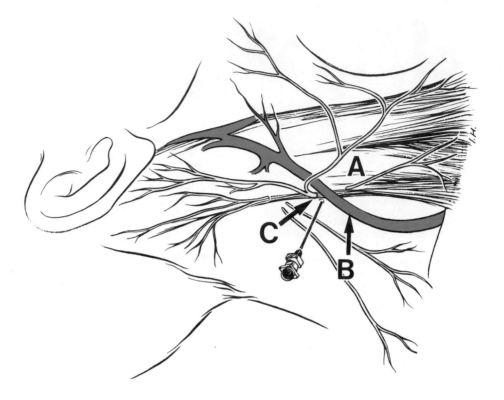

Figure 1-2. Superficial cervical plexus block: Anatomic drawing showing the sternocleidomastoid muscle **A,** the external jugular vein **B,** and the superficial cervical plexus **C.**

cervical transverse process is marked. A line is drawn from this point to the suprasternal notch. A point 1.5 cm caudal to the tip of the mastoid is marked along this line. This overlies the tip of the transverse process of the second cervical vertebra. Points marked 1.5 and 3 cm below this point indicate the transverse processes of C3 and C4 respectively (Fig. 1-4).

Technique

One and one-half inch, 22-gauge needles are inserted to a depth of 1.5–2 cm perpendicular to all planes of the skin to contact the respective transverse processes. Paresthesias may or may not be elicited. Three ml of local anesthetic are then injected at each site following negative aspiration for blood or cerebrospinal fluid. If needles are properly placed, onset of analgesia will occur within 5 minutes regardless of the drug

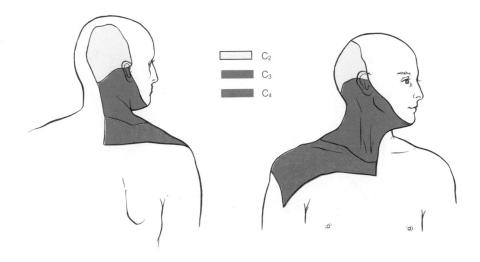

Figure 1-3. Superficial cervical plexus block—distribution of cutaneous anesthesia.

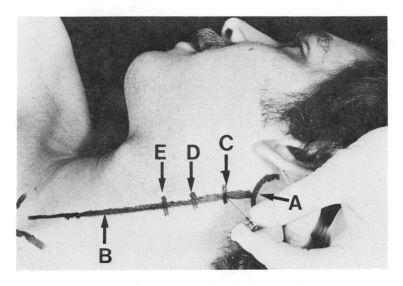

Figure 1-4. Deep cervical plexus block: **A** indicates the tip of the mastoid process, **B** a line drawn from that point to the suprasternal notch, **C** the site for injection of C2, and **D** and **E** the sites for injection of C3 and C4 respectively.

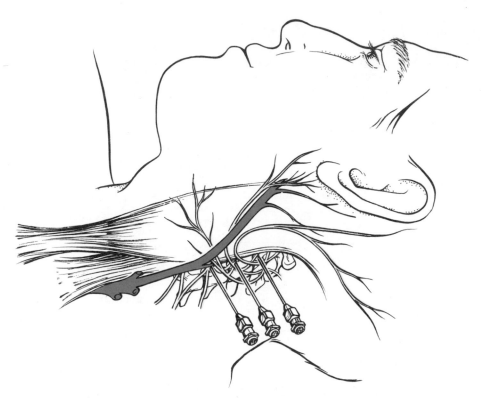

Figure 1-5. Deep cervical plexus block—anatomic drawing: The needles (from right to left) are noted at the sulci of the transverse processes of C2, C3 and C4.

used (Fig. 1-5). The area of cutaneous anesthesia is the same as for superficial cervical block (Fig. 1-3), but deeper structures are anesthetized as well.

COMPLICATIONS

An infrequent, but possible, complication of superficial cervical plexus block is accidental injection into the internal jugular vein. If intravascular injection of a large bolus of drug occurs, systemic toxicity may result. Tears in the wall of the vein can lead to hematoma formation. If penetration of the vein occurs with a needle unattached to a syringe, the possibility of air embolism exists.

The most common complication of deep cervical block is recurrent laryngeal nerve paralysis followed closely in frequency of incidence by production of a stellate ganglion block and respiratory distress. These are transient complications, and only of significance if bilateral interruption of the recurrent laryngeal nerve occurs. In this situation, endotracheal intubation is mandatory.

Bilateral stellate ganglion block may result in profound bradycardia due to interruption of cardioaccelerator fibers.

Less frequently, a nerve root sleeve may be entered and injection of local anesthetic will produce a cervical subarachnoid block with possible phrenic nerve block. The other structure of major importance in the area is the vertebral artery. Injection into the vertebral artery will result in convulsions or apnea with as little as 0.5 ml of local anesthetic because of its direct flow to the brain stem. If colloidal materials such as depot steroids are added to local anesthetics for pain management, injection of this material into the vertebral artery will result in Wallenberg's syndrome, occlusion of the posterior inferior cerebellar artery. ■

2

Brachial Plexus Block

INTERSCALENE APPROACH

Interscalene block is the preferred technique for shoulder and upper arm surgery, but increased volumes of local anesthetic drugs are required to obtain anesthesia of the forearm and hand. As with all brachial plexus blocks, anesthesia of the medial upper arm requires blockade of the intercostobrachial nerve (See Axillary Approach, in this chapter).

The more distal the injection from the point of origin of the nerves composing the brachial plexus, the slower the onset of block. Interscalene block can be expected to be complete in approximately 10 minutes, whereas axillary block may take as long as 25 minutes. To hasten the onset of anesthesia, peripheral blocks either at the elbow or wrist may be performed in conjunction with axillary block.

Anatomy

The cervical nerves of C5 to T1 leave their respective intervertebral foramina and pass in the sulci of the transverse processes laterally and caudad between the anterior and medial scalene muscles which are

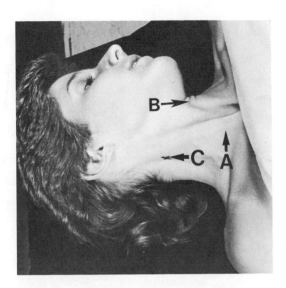

Figure 2-1. Brachial plexus block—interscalene approach: **A** indicates the posterior border of the sternocleidomastoid muscle, **B** the cricoid cartilage, and **C** the interscalene groove. The needle is inserted at point **C** and directed 45° caudad and medial to the planes of the skin until paresthesias are obtained or the transverse process of C6 is contacted.

attached to the anterior and posterior tubercles of the transverse processes. The space between these two muscles is known as the interscalene groove and contains all of the cervical nerve roots.

Landmarks

The patient is placed supine with the head rotated to the side opposite that to be blocked. The shoulder on the block side is depressed. The patient is then requested to lift the head to identify the posterior border of the sternocleidomastoid muscle. The index finger is placed on the sternocleidomastoid muscle, then rolled posterolaterally over the anterior scalene to fall into the interscalene groove at a level opposite the cricothyroid notch (C6 level) (Fig. 2-1).

Technique

A 1.5-inch, 22-gauge short bevel needle is introduced perpendicular to all planes of the skin at the tip of the palpating finger and directed approximately 45° caudad until paresthesias are obtained as the needle enters the interscalene groove or until the transverse process of C6 is contacted (Fig. 2-2). After negative aspiration, 25 ml of local anesthetic

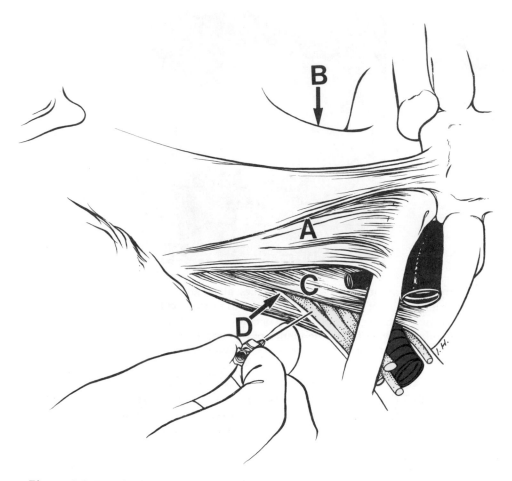

Figure 2-2. Brachial plexus block—interscalene approach: Anatomic drawing showing the sternocleidomastoid muscle, **(A)** the level of the cricoid cartilage **(B),** the anterior scalene muscle **(C),** and the interscalene groove **(D).**

are injected. Anesthesia encompasses the shoulder and the upper extremity to just below the elbow with this volume of solution (Fig. 2-3). Forty ml of anesthetic will usually anesthetize the entire arm with the possible exception of that portion supplied by the ulnar nerve.

SUPRACLAVICULAR APPROACH

The supraclavicular approach will produce anesthesia of the entire upper arm, forearm and hand, but will spare a portion of the shoulder.

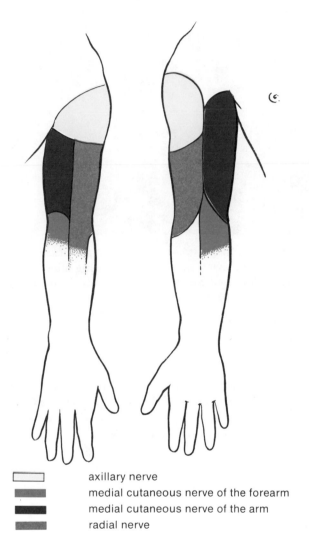

axillary nerve
medial cutaneous nerve of the forearm
medial cutaneous nerve of the arm
radial nerve

Figure 2-3. Brachial plexus block—interscalene approach, distribution of cutaneous anesthesia: Brachial plexus block with 25 ml of local anesthetic will anesthetize the shoulder and upper arm but will spare portions of the forearm and hand, particularly the ulnar distribution. Volumes of up to 40 ml are required to anesthetize the entire extremity.

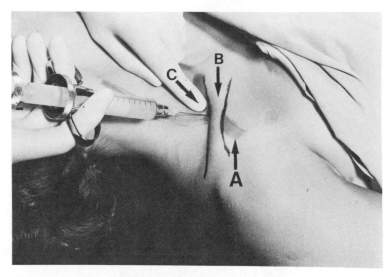

Figure 2-4. Brachial plexus block—supraclavicular approach: **A** indicates the subclavian artery, **B** the clavicle, and **C** the palpating finger on the first rib lateral to the artery. The needle is advanced to contact the first rib following which local anesthetic is injected.

Anatomy

As the cervical nerve roots pass between the scalene muscles, they divide to form component parts of the brachial plexus which unite in a bundle that passes caudad to lie on the first rib lateral to the subclavian artery at about the midpoint of the clavicle.

Landmarks

The subclavian artery is palpated on the first rib just 1–2 cm cephalad to the midpoint of the clavicle and the brachial plexus is palpated lateral to the artery (Fig. 2-4).

Technique

A 1.5 in., 22-gauge needle is introduced lateral to the pulsating subclavian artery to contact the first rib. Paresthesias in the hand or forearm may be obtained. On withdrawing the needle slightly from contact with the rib, 25–30 ml of local anesthetic are injected after negative aspiration (Fig. 2-5). In the event the artery is not palpable because of obesity or heavy musculature, the midpoint of the clavicle should be located and the needle inserted at a point 2 cm cephalad to

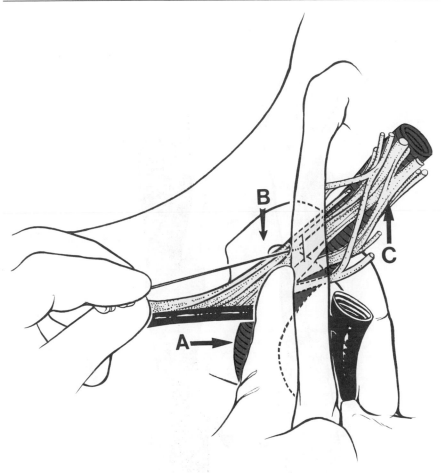

Figure 2-5. Brachial plexus block—supraclavicular approach: Anatomic drawing showing the subclavian artery **(A),** the first rib **(B),** and the brachial plexus **(C).**

that point and directed caudad until paresthesias are elicited or the first rib is contacted. Anesthesia produced by supraclavicular brachial plexus block is shown in Figure 2-6.

AXILLARY APPROACH

This block is usually preferred for procedures involving the hand. It is also very useful in anesthetizing the forearm and elbow, but anesthesia of the distribution of the musculocutaneous nerve (the lateral forearm) is sometimes incomplete. Axillary blocks are relatively easy to perform and have few complications.

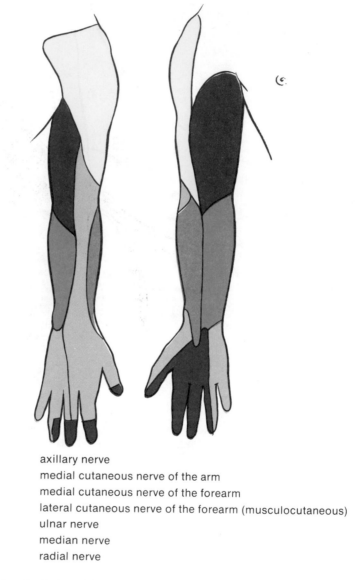

axillary nerve
medial cutaneous nerve of the arm
medial cutaneous nerve of the forearm
lateral cutaneous nerve of the forearm (musculocutaneous)
ulnar nerve
median nerve
radial nerve

Figure 2-6. Brachial plexus block—supraclavicular approach: Cutaneous distribution of anesthesia with the supraclavicular approach. 25 ml of local anesthetic will anesthetize the entire upper extremity including the shoulder.

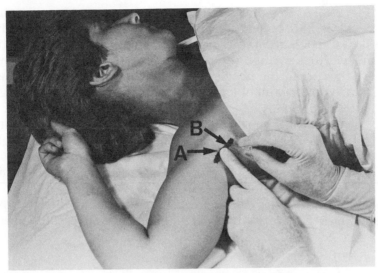

Figure 2-7. Brachial plexus block—axillary approach: **A** indicates the palpable axillary artery and **B** the needle directed toward the artery at the apex of the axilla until the "click" of the fascial sheath is felt or paresthesias are obtained. At that point, the local anesthetic is injected. If the artery is pierced, the needle is advanced through the sheath to contact the humerus and then withdrawn slightly before injection.

Anatomy

As the brachial plexus passes under the clavicle and travels caudad to the axilla, it is contained within a fascial compartment, the axillary sheath. In the sheath, the ulnar nerve is posterior to the axillary artery, the radial nerve posterior and lateral, and the median nerve anterior. The medial brachial cutaneous and medial antebracheal cutaneous nerves are medial to the artery as well.

Landmarks

With the patient in the supine position, the arm is abducted to 90° with the forearm supinated and resting on the table above the patient's head. The axillary artery is palpated as high in the apex of the axilla as is possible, usually under the insertion of the pectoralis major into the humerus (Fig. 2-7).

Technique

With the operator's index finger on the axillary artery, a 1.5 in., 22-gauge, short bevel needle is inserted through the skin perpendicular to all planes directly toward the artery until the "click" of the fascial sheath is felt (Fig. 2-8). At this time, with both hands removed from the patient, if the needle is in the sheath, it will remain in a position perpendicular to the skin and pulsations may be noted. If these findings obtain, tubing is connected to a syringe reservoir of local anesthetic or the syringe itself is attached to the needle which is held firmly to avoid displacement. Thirty to forty ml of local anesthetic are injected following aspiration after each 5 ml.

In the event that arterial puncture occurs simultaneously with the "click" of the fascia, the needle may be passed directly through the artery until blood can no longer be aspirated. The needle is then withdrawn approximately 0.5 cm, and after negative aspiration the volume of local anesthetic can be injected at this site.

Some anesthesiologists recommend seeking paresthesias of each of the major nerve trucks in order to guarantee successful block, but

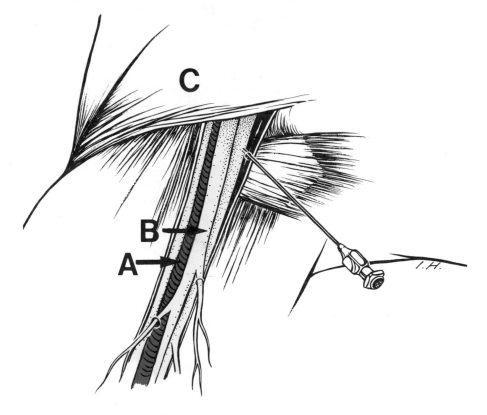

Figure 2-8. Brachial plexus block—axillary approach: Anatomic drawing showing the axillary artery **(A)**, the brachial plexus within the axillary sheath **(B)**, and the pectoralis major muscle **(C)**.

the incidence of postblock neuralgias is increased when paresthesias are obtained.

If the solution is properly introduced into the axillary sheath, a "sausage" will form in the axilla following the axis of the humerus. In the event that the solution is injected outside of the sheath, a conical-shaped elevation of the tissues will develop with the apex at the site of the needle insertion. If block is performed adequately high in the axilla rather than at the point of insertion of the pectoralis into the humerus, it is unnecessary to block the musculocutaneous nerve separately. As the needle is removed from the sheath, 5 ml of local anesthetic are injected subcutaneously in a line perpendicular to and overlying the sheath to block the intercostobrachial and medial cutaneous nerves of the forearm.

Upon completion of the block, the arm is placed at the patient's side and digital pressure is exerted just distal to the injection site to encourage proximal spread of the anesthetic. If the axillary artery has been punctured, then pressure is exerted over the puncture site to prevent hematoma formation. Onset of block can be determined by evidence of rapidly developing weakness of the triceps and by the appearance of venous dilation of the extremity due to sympathectomy. The extent of anesthesia is shown in Figure 2-9.

Complications

The interscalene approach to the brachial plexus carries with it the same risks as deep cervical plexus block; i.e., recurrent laryngeal nerve paralysis, stellate ganglion block, phrenic block, subarachnoid block, and intravascular injection with systemic toxicity. There is the additional risk of pneumothorax, particularly when the interscalene block is performed on the right side. Perforation of the thoracic duct on the left has also been reported.

The most common complication of the supraclavicular approach is pneumothorax due to perforation of the cupola of the pleura. This is most readily avoided by maintaining pressure over the subclavian artery on the first rib as the needle is inserted lateral to the palpating finger. Pneumothorax of less than 25%, when it occurs, generally requires no therapy. Pneumothorax in excess of 25% will require closed drainage.

The axillary approach to the brachial plexus produces the least complications. The major difficulty arises with continued probing of the sheath to identify through paresthesias the major nerve trunks to the extremity. Prolonged paresthesias and sensory deficits have been reported to be higher with individual nerve identification as compared to the fascial "click" or axillary artery penetration as identifying techniques for the axillary sheath.

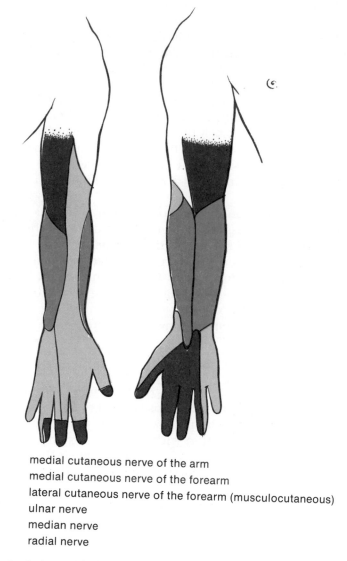

medial cutaneous nerve of the arm
medial cutaneous nerve of the forearm
lateral cutaneous nerve of the forearm (musculocutaneous)
ulnar nerve
median nerve
radial nerve

Figure 2-9. Brachial plexus block—axillary approach: Distribution of cutaneous anesthesia. The entire arm and forearm are anesthetized but the shoulder is spared.

Pressure of large volumes of local anesthetic injected into the sheath dissipates rapidly and is of no significance in producing postinjection neurologic deficits. ■

3

Lumbar Plexus Block

The lumbar plexus gives off the nerves which innervate the anterior and medial aspects of the leg. An alternative to blocking them separately, is to anesthetize them with a single injection if desired. In combination with blockade of the sciatic nerve, which arises partially from the sacral plexus, anesthesia of the entire leg can be obtained.

Anatomy

The lumbar plexus is formed by the anterior rami of the first four lumbar nerves and may include branches from the 12th thoracic and 5th lumbar as well. As in the cervical region, these nerves are contained within a fascial compartment which then follows the major nerves to the lower extremity. As the lumbar plexus forms at the transverse processes of the lumbar vertebrae, the nerves lie deep in the substance of the psoas major muscle and, after passing through the muscle, form the lateral femoral cutaneous, femoral and obturator nerves which pass caudad to supply innervation to the lower extremity. It is at the point just before the nerves enter the psoas muscle that the fascial compartment containing these fibers may be entered to perform the lumbar paravertebral somatic block.

PARAVERTEBRAL APPROACH

Landmarks

The patient is placed in the prone position with a pillow under the abdomen to increase the distance between the lower ribs and the iliac crest by decreasing the lumbar curve. A line is drawn connecting the tips of the lumbar spines. A second line is drawn parallel and 8 cm lateral to the line connecting the spines. The point where this second line intersects the crest of the ilium is marked. If points 2.5 cm apart are marked cephalad from this point along the line, they will serve as points of entry for the lumbar plexus, with the lowest mark at the crest of the ilium the point of entry for L5 (Fig. 3-1).

Technique

A 3.5-inch, 22-gauge spinal needle is inserted through skin wheals opposite the nerves to be blocked and directed 45° medial and 45° caudad to a depth of approximately 3 inches. At this point, bone is contacted and paresthesias elicited. This indicates entry into the sheath.

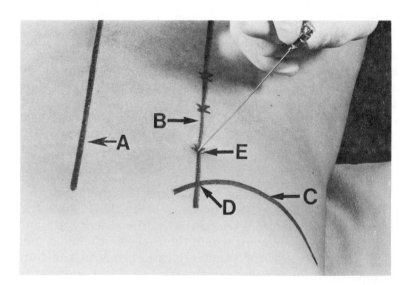

Figure 3-1. Lumbar plexus block—paravertebral approach: A line **A** is drawn connecting the spinous processes of the lumbar vertebrae. A second line **B** is drawn 8 cm lateral to line A. **C** is the crest of the ilium. Where line **B** intersects line **C** at point **D** is the site of insertion of the needle for the L5 nerve root. **E** indicates the needle directed 45° medial and 45° caudad at a point 2.5 cm cephalad from point **D** to block the 4th lumbar nerve root.

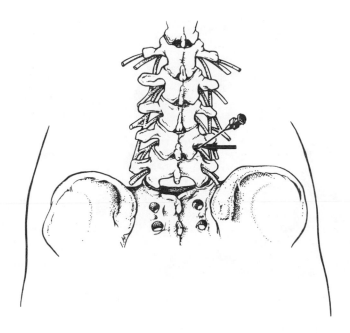

Figure 3-2. Lumbar plexus block—paravertebral approach: Anatomic drawing with arrow showing nerve roots exiting respective intervertebral foramina.

A large volume of 35—40 ml of local anesthetic may be injected to block the entire lumbar and sacral plexuses, or smaller volumes of 3—5 ml at multiple sites will block the lumbar nerves as they exit from their respective intervertebral foramina (Fig. 3-2).

Anesthesia produced with the complete lumbosacral paravertebral block will include the entire lower extremity. The volume used will determine the extent to which the block develops distally.

INGUINAL PARAVASCULAR TECHNIQUE

Anatomy

This technique utilizes the fascial compartment around the femoral nerve to carry injected anesthetic solution to the area of formation of the lumbar plexus.

Landmarks

With the patient in the supine position, a skin wheal is raised lateral to the femoral artery just caudal to the inguinal ligament (Fig. 3-3).

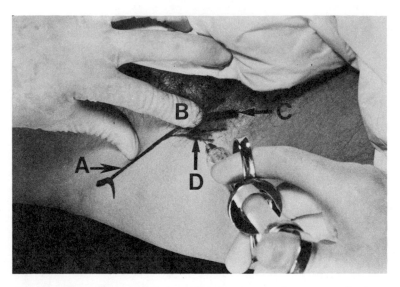

Figure 3-3. Lumbar plexus block—inguinal paravascular approach: **A** indicates the inguinal ligament, **B** the palpating finger on the femoral artery, **C** the femoral vein, and **D** the point of needle insertion for the sheath containing the femoral nerve. The needle is inserted in a cephalad direction to enter the femoral canal. As local anesthetic is injected, the sheath is compressed distally to force the anesthetic up into the fascial compartment containing the lumbar plexus.

Technique

With a finger placed on the artery, a 22-gauge, 1.5-inch, short bevel needle is inserted just lateral to the palpating finger in a cephalad direction seeking paresthesias of the femoral nerve. When these are obtained, a 40-ml bolus of local anesthetic is injected while pressure is maintained distal to the point of insertion of the needle to force the solution up into the lumbar area (Fig. 3-4).

COMPLICATIONS

With the blind technique utilized in the paravertebral approach to the lumbar plexus, the needle must be placed in close proximity to the intervertebral foramen. This raises the possibility of penetration of a nerve root sleeve or of the dura itself with consequent subarachnoid block on injection. Often, when the needle reaches the foramen, paresthesias are elicited. The needle should then be withdrawn slightly so that intraneural injection does not occur. Pressure of the solution intraneurally may produce transient or permanent neurological deficits.

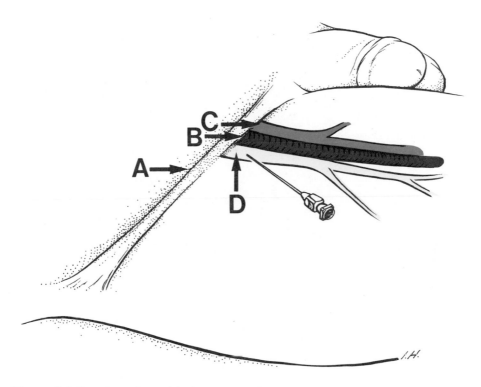

Figure 3-4. Lumbar plexus block—inguinal paravascular approach: Anatomic drawing showing relationship of inguinal ligament **A** to femoral artery **B,** femoral vein **C,** and femoral sheath **D** containing the femoral nerve.

The inguinal paravascular approach to the lumbar plexus requires a large volume of local anesthetic. Problems in supplementation of the block can occur with the maximal drug dosage having already been administered. Intravascular or retroperitoneal injection can also occur if the needle is not accurately placed within the femoral sheath. ■

Section II

Neural Axis Blocks

4

Subarachnoid Block

Spinal (subarachnoid) blockade is the oldest form of anesthesia that is still practiced. It is most commonly used for surgical procedures below the umbilicus (T10). The ease of this technique combined with its safety, rapidity of onset, and high reliability make this one of the most widely practiced forms of regional anesthesia in use today.

Anatomy

Lumbar puncture is performed by placing a needle through one of the intervertebral spaces from L2 to the sacrum. The spinal cord terminates at the level of L1 while the dural sac ends at S2. Therefore, below L1, the subarachnoid space contains only the nerve roots of the cauda equina floating in cerebrospinal fluid (CSF). In the common midline approach several structures are encountered by the needle in its passage to the subarachnoid space (Fig. 4-1). Beneath the skin lies a usually thin layer of subcutaneous fat which overlies the supraspinous ligament. Deep to this ligament is the spongy interspinous ligament and deep to this is the very tough ligamentum flavum. The epidural space lies between the ligamentum flavum and the dural sac and is described in greater detail in the following chapter (Epidural Block).

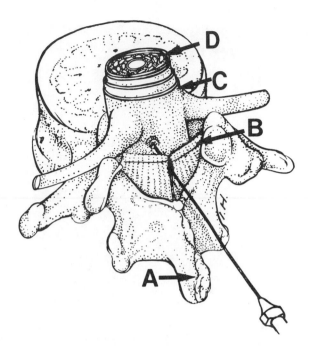

Figure 4-1. Spinal canal: Anatomic drawing of the spinal canal and its contents. **A** represents the spinous process, **B** the ligamentum flavum, **C** the dura mater, and **D** the cauda equina.

The spinal meninges are encountered next and consist of the dura mater, which is separated from the arachnoid by a very thin layer of serous fluid which can form a potential space (the subdural space). Deep to the arachnoid lies the subarachnoid space which contains CSF, the weblike trabeculations of the pia mater, and the nerve roots of the cauda equina.

Landmarks

The most common needle entry site is the interspace between the L3 and L4 spinous processes. This is located by palpating the highest level of the iliac crests and drawing a line between them, known as the intercristal line, which overlies the L4 spinous process; or if the patient is well flexed forward, the line may overlie the L4-5 interspace (Fig. 4-2). The midline of the back is found by palpating the spinous processes.

MOST COMMON TECHNIQUE (HYPERBARIC)

Midline Approach

The patient is placed in the lateral position with the side to be operated on dependent. The table is adjusted so that the patient's spine is parallel with the floor. An assistant should remain available to keep

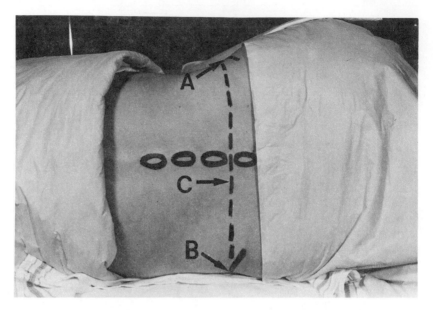

Figure 4-2. Subarachnoid block—landmarks: **A** and **B** indicate the right and left iliac crests, respectively, and **C** the intercristal line which overlies the L4-5 interspace. Lumbar puncture is performed preferably at this interspace to avoid injuring the spinal cord, which may extend caudally as far as L3.

the patient in as much forward flexion as possible. This separates the spinous processes, opens up the interspace, and insures that the patient is prevented from falling. If a difficult block is anticipated due to the patient's obesity, the block should be done with the patient in the sitting position with his feet supported on a stool and the assistant standing squarely in front of the patient. This greatly facilitates finding the midline. A sterile drape is placed under the patient such that any spilled prep solution will not fall upon the sheets of the operating table. The most easily palpated interspace below the L2 spinous process is selected, usually L3-4, and a small skin wheal is produced with local anesthetic. The spinal needle (see the section Spinal Needles in this chapter) is placed in the middle of the interspace, parallel to the sagittal plane, and angled 10° cephalad (Fig. 4-3). One hand palpates the interspace while the other inserts the needle until the supraspinous ligament is entered as is demonstrated by the needle's maintaining its position when released. The needle is then grasped in the two-handed position (Fig. 4-4) which maximizes tactile feedback and minimizes needle bending. With the bevel of the needle (indicated by the notch in the hub) directed toward the patient's side so as to spread rather than

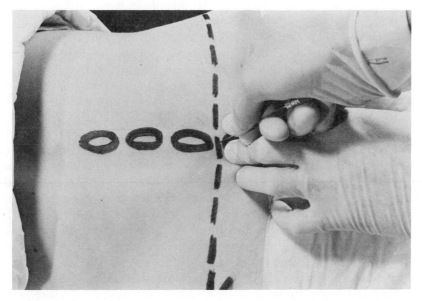

Figure 4-3. Subarachnoid block: Inserting spinal needle into interspace L4-5. One hand palpates the interspace while the other controls the needle during insertion into the supraspinous ligament.

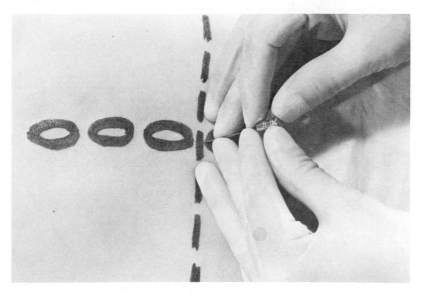

Figure 4-4. Subarachnoid block: Correct technique for advancing spinal needle. The two-handed position maximizes tactile feedback and provides excellent control of a flexible needle.

cut the longitudinal dural fibers, the needle is then advanced slowly toward the subarachnoid space. Some increased resistance will be noticed as the needle traverses the ligamentum flavum, particularly when large bore needles are used. A "pop" can often be felt as the dura and arachnoid are pierced. These characteristic sensations are subject to a great deal of variation, particularly in the elderly or the parturient patient. The greater the experience of the operator, the more clues he will have as to the position of the needle tip.

The stylet is then removed and the hub is observed for the free flow of CSF. This may take several seconds when a 25–26 gauge needle is used. It is often helpful, even if CSF appears in the hub of a small bore needle, to attach a 3 ml syringe to ascertain whether fluid can be readily aspirated. If free flow is not obtained, the needle tip is repositioned slightly (see the section Common Problems in this chapter). When free flow is obtained, the needle is rotated 90° and 180° and, if flow is still present, the local anesthetic is then injected over 5–10 seconds with the hub held firmly in the thumb and index finger while the back of the hand is securely placed against the patient's back (Fig. 4-5) such that needle movement is prevented. CSF should be aspirated before, at the half-way point, and after injection of the anesthetic to demonstrate that

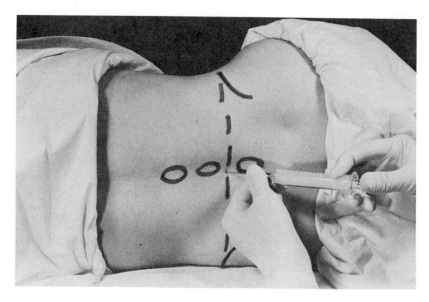

Figure 4-5. Subarachnoid block: Stabilizing needle during injection of anesthetic. The fingers of the left hand grasp the needle hub while the back of the hand rests securely against the patient's back. The needle is thus held immobile while the anesthetic is being injected.

the needle has not moved out of position. The needle is then removed and the patient placed in the desired position to allow the block to set up. If, for example, the right leg is to be operated on, the patient should be kept in the right lateral decubitus position until the onset of sensory block is established, usually within 2–4 minutes, before the patient is positioned for surgery. If the level of anesthesia at 2 and 5 minutes indicates that the block is either too high or low, then the table may be adjusted to take advantage of the hyperbaricity (heaviness) of the solution. Lowering the head of the table will tend to raise the level of the block.

The blood pressure is checked every 30 seconds for the first 5 minutes and at least every minute until the level of the block has stabilized, and then every 5 minutes thereafter. At the first sign of a drop in blood pressure, it should be checked even more frequently until the nature of the change is clearly defined. The EKG is monitored continuously and the level of the block is determined at 2, 5, 10 and 20 minutes after the local anesthetic injection. The highest level of blockade should be recorded so that for subsequent spinal anesthetics the dose can be fine tuned to perfection.

VARIATIONS IN TECHNIQUES

Paramedian Approach

This technique is very useful since it does not depend on the patient's ability to flex the spine. Approaching the subarachnoid space from the side avoids contact with the spinous processes as well as the supra- and interspinous ligaments which are sometimes heavily calcified and difficult to traverse. The landmarks are the same as for the midline approach except that the needle entry point is a thumb breadth lateral to the center of the interspace. With the patient in the lateral position, the entry point is on the dependent side of the patient. The needle is angled 10° cephalad as in the midline approach, but it is also angled 20° toward the midline. If bone is encountered during advancement of the needle, it is most likely on a lamina. Redirecting the tip in a more cephalad and medial direction and then walking off the lamina will result in correct placement (Fig. 4-6).

Taylor Approach

This is a variation of the paramedian approach except that the L5-S1 interspace is entered. The landmark used is the posterior superior iliac spine. A skin wheal is placed one thumb breadth cephalad and

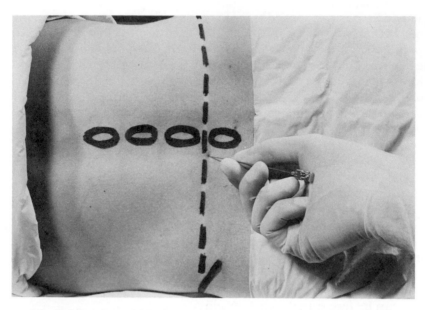

Figure 4-6. Subarachnoid block—paramedian approach: The needle is inserted one thumb breadth lateral from the midline of the interspace on the dependent side and directed 10° cephalad and 20° medially to drop into the subarachnoid space. If a lamina is contacted, the needle is walked off bone in a cephalad direction.

medial to this bony prominence and the needle directed approximately 45° cephalad and medial. If bone is encountered, the needle is redirected cephalad and medial until it can be walked off into the intervertebral space (Fig. 4-7).

Saddle Block

When anesthesia of only the perineum (lower sacral roots) is desired, a small dose of hyperbaric local anesthetic may be injected with the patient in the sitting position. The patient is kept sitting until the block has adequately set up, usually about 5 minutes. Hypotension, nausea, and other side effects of spinal anesthesia are seldom seen with this technique. Local anesthetic doses are one-half those for a T10 level; i.e., lidocaine 25 mg or tetracaine 4 mg.

Hypobaric Spinal

The specific gravity of CSF is usually in the range of 1.003–1.009. A 0.1% solution of tetracaine can be prepared by diluting 10 mg of tetracaine in 9 ml of distilled water; this solution is hypobaric when

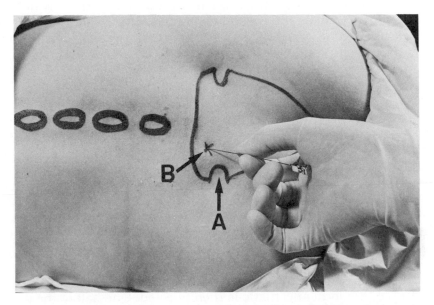

Figure 4-7. Subarachnoid block—Taylor approach: **A** indicates the posterior superior iliac spine. The needle entry site, **B,** is one thumb breadth cephalad and medial to **A.** The needle is directed 45° cephalad and medial to enter the dural sac at the L5-S1 interspace.

injected into the subarachnoid space. This means that it will tend to rise to the highest point when injected as opposed to hyperbaric anesthetic solutions, which tend to settle to the lowest point. The technique is most useful for procedures performed in the prone or jackknife positions, usually procedures involving the back or rectum. It is also useful for lower extremity surgery when the patient is to be placed in the lateral position with the surgical site upward.

If the needle is to be placed with the patient in the prone position, the paramedian approach is easiest since the patient cannot fully flex the spine. The dose of local anesthetic is the same as in the hyperbaric technique but the duration of anesthesia is less since a much larger volume is injected, providing a lower anesthetic concentration, and hence, a thinner block which regresses faster. After injection of the hypobaric solution the patient should be placed in a slight head down position to avoid a high level of anesthesia.

Isobaric Spinal

Tetracaine 1% solution is isobaric at body temperature, and for this reason, when injected into the subarachnoid space, will not move with changes in patient position. Six mg mixed with 4 ml of CSF will provide an L1 level of anesthesia when injected. The variability of CSF specific gravity makes the possibility of obtaining a slightly hypo- or hyperbaric solution possible and provides an element of unpredictability with the technique.

Continuous Spinal

As with any continuous technique in which a catheter is utilized, this procedure has the advantage of allowing the dose of local anesthetic to be titrated to achieve and then maintain any desired level of anesthesia. Any approach to the subarachnoid space can be used. A Tuohy epidural needle with a Huber point, as is usually found in disposable continuous epidural kits, is advanced with the bevel directed laterally until free-flowing CSF is obtained. The bevel is then directed cephalad and a plastic catheter is placed through the needle, 2 cm beyond the needle tip. The needle is withdrawn, and the catheter taped in place as described in Chapter 5, Epidural Block. CSF should be aspirated through the catheter to demonstrate proper position and patency of the catheter, whereupon the local anesthetic is then injected. One-half of the usual dose given for a "single shot" spinal is given initially. Top-up doses are usually one-half of the initial dose. It should be remembered that the dead space of the standard epidural catheter is about 0.25 ml, which assumes importance since small volumes of anesthetic are injected. This technique is usually limited to the elderly population since the use of a very large bore epidural needle almost always produces a spinal headache in a young person.

COMMON PROBLEMS

1. *Bone is encountered during midline approach.* Usually the problem is that the needle tip is not in the midline. A handy way to determine which way to redirect the needle is to ask the patient to localize the discomfort caused by the needle, and then reposition accordingly. The bone should be walked off in the appropriate direction. If the needle position cannot be localized, then blindly walking off bone in all four directions will often allow correct placement. The patient's position should be checked to be sure that he is maximally flexed with knees to chin to maximally open the interspinous space. If the patient cannot flex his spine adequately or all other maneuvers fail, then the paramedian approach will often prove successful. Occasionally, particularly in older people, the ligaments are calcified enough to feel almost like bone except that with moderate pressure the needle will advance slowly.

2. *A paresthesia is obtained.* If CSF flows readily and the paresthesia was fleeting, then injection of anesthetic can be safely done. A paresthesia during injection necessitates that the needle be repositioned before any further drug is injected. If CSF is not obtained, the paresthesia should be localized by the patient to serve as a guide in repositioning the needle, i.e., a paresthesia to the right hip indicates that the needle should be directed to the patient's left side.

3. *Blood appears in the hub.* If the initial flow of CSF is bloody but then clears, injection of the anesthetic may be performed. If it does not clear, this may indicate a recent subarachnoid hemorrhage which is a relative contraindication to injection of local anesthetic.

4. *CSF appears in the hub but cannot be aspirated easily.* If first rotating the needle and then repositioning it in and out a few millimeters does not solve the problem then, as long as CSF continues to flow from the hub, injection of the anesthetic will usually provide good anesthesia. This problem is encountered most often in the elderly.

ANESTHETIC LEVELS REQUIRED FOR SURGERY

For surgery of the lower extremities, perineum, and bladder, a T10 level is required. One exception to this is procedures involving the testes, which have descended from the abdomen, and require a T4 level. Surgical procedures on the lower abdomen such as appendectomy, herniorrhaphy, or hysterectomy also require a T4 level. Upper abdominal procedures are better performed under general anesthesia.

Table 4–1 indicates onset and duration for various local anesthetics. Doses are approximated for the patient of average stature. Shorter

Table 4-1
Use of Local Anesthetics (in Hyperbaric Dextrose)* for Surgery

Drug	Dose (in mg)		Onset (min)	Duration (min)	
	T10	T4		Plain	With Epinephrine (0.2 mg)
Procaine, 5%	125	175	5	30–45	60–75
Lidocaine, 5%	50	100	4	45–60	60–90
Tetracaine, 0.5%	8	14	2	60–90	120–180

*Hyperbaric procaine and tetracaine are prepared by combining a 10% procaine or 1% tetracaine solution in a 1:1 mixture with 10% dextrose solution. Lidocaine is usually supplied premixed in a 7.5% dextrose solution.

patients will require proportionally lower doses and taller patients, higher doses. Markedly obese patients require lower dosages for their height. In the pregnant female at term, the dose for cesarean section is reduced one-third such that tetracaine 6–8 mg will produce the desired T4 level.

The addition of epinephrine to prolong the effect of the local anesthetic is slightly controversial. The placement of a vasoconstrictor into the subarachnoid space may, it is argued, compromise blood supply to the spinal cord. No clear evidence has arisen to substantiate this fear, however.

SPINAL NEEDLES

Several sizes and styles of needles are available (Fig. 4-8), but the 3.5-inch Quincke-Babcock needle (cutting edge, medium bevel) is the standard choice. Two sizes are commonly used: 25–26-gauge, to be used in patients under 50 years of age, and 22-gauge, to be used in older patients. The reason for this is that the main complication of subarachnoid block in the younger population is spinal headache, the incidence of which is decreased by the use of smaller diameter needles. In older patients, the incidence of headache is much less, but the difficulty in placing a thin and flimsy needle through often heavily calcified ligaments can be great. Therefore the larger diameter, stiffer needle is preferable. Twenty-five- and 26-gauge needles are usually used with an introducer needle (Fig. 4-8) which is placed into the interspinous ligament and serves as a guide for the smaller needle, which is then inserted through it.

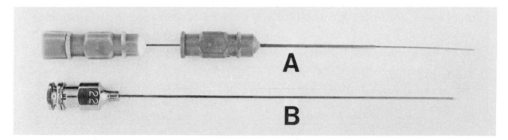

Figure 4-8. Spinal needles: A 25-gauge Quincke-Babcock (Monoject, St. Louis, MO) needle **(A)** is shown inserted through a large gauge introducer needle. The introducer needle is first inserted into the interspace to pass beyond the ligamentum flavum. The 25-gauge needle is then threaded through the larger needle to penetrate the dura. **B** indicates the standard 22-gauge Quincke-Babcock (Monoject) spinal needle.

CONTRAINDICATIONS

These include infection at the needle entry site, severe blood loss or shock, significant coagulopathy, septicemia, and patient refusal. Progressive neurologic disease may be a relative contraindication. Each case must be evaluated individually.

COMPLICATIONS

The most common complication or side effect of subarachnoid block is hypotension secondary to sympathectomy. Nausea may be the first sign of hypotension, but usually it occurs in the presence of a normal blood pressure. It is more likely due to unopposed vagal tone with gut contraction and sphincter relaxation following sympathectomy.

Postdural puncture headache is the most annoying of the complications of subarachnoid block. Headache is due to leakage of spinal fluid into the epidural space with the subsequent low CSF pressure contributing to traction on cerebral vessels. Transient neurological sequelae are rare since the introduction of small caliber spinal needles and the use of modern equipment and drugs. Each of these complications will be discussed in further detail in Section VI, Complications.

BENEFITS

Evidence of decreased blood loss, a lower incidence of thrombophlebitis, and decreased mortality using subarachnoid block versus general anesthesia have been reported in studies of total hip replacement procedures. Monitoring of CNS function in the awake patient provides an added margin of safety in transurethral resection of the prostate (TURP), since the first signs of water intoxication are disorientation, nausea, and restlessness. Generally, the minimal physiologic disturbances of a T10 spinal level of anesthesia offer many advantages in patients with multiple system disease. ■

5

Epidural Block

Lumbar epidural anesthesia, which is the most commonly used form of this technique, has many of the same indications as does spinal block. They are both used for any abdominal surgical procedure, preferably below the umbilicus. Placement of a catheter into the epidural space at any level from sacrum to the cervical region allows continuous, controllable levels of anesthesia of most areas of the body. This, combined with the avoidance of spinal headache, has made the technique increasingly popular, especially for obstetric labor and delivery.

Anatomy

The triangularly shaped epidural space lies between the tough ligamentum flavum and the dura. It is in continuity from the sacral hiatus to the base of the skull and varies in anteroposterior (AP) diameter at different sites, being greatest at the midline. The greatest AP diameter is found in the lumbar area (4–6 mm) tapering to 2 mm in the cervical area. The lumbar epidural space is the easiest and safest to approach for this reason because of the large interlaminar space and the fact that inadvertent dural puncture would be below the end of the spinal cord.

The lumbar approach should be thoroughly mastered before attempting the procedure at higher levels. The thoracic and cervical epidural spaces can be approached most easily between T10-12 and C7-T1 respectively because the interlaminal and epidural spaces are relatively larger at these levels. The spinous processes at the midthoracic levels are caudad to the next lower vertebral bodies, requiring a paramedian approach in an extremely cephalad direction if the epidural space is to be entered at these levels.

The epidural space contains fat and a plexus of valveless veins which lie primarily in the lateral aspect of the space. These provide venous drainage from the spinal cord into the azygos vein and can serve as an alternate pathway for pelvic venous drainage when obstruction of the inferior vena cava occurs as in pregnancy.

CERVICAL EPIDURAL BLOCK

This technique can be used for surgical anesthesia for neck surgery (carotid endarterectomy, thyroidectomy or in pain management). Only sensory blocking concentrations should be used, however, to avoid blocking the phrenic nerve which arises from the fourth and fifth cervical nerves. Motor blockade could result in respiratory compromise.

In the cervical and thoracic regions the minimum distance between the ligamentum flavum and the dura and the strongly negative pressure in the epidural space makes the use of the hanging drop technique preferable. The use of a winged needle facilitates manipulation during needle introduction into the epidural space. Figure 5-1 shows the conventional Tuohy and the Weiss winged needles.

Landmarks

The patient is placed in the sitting position with head and neck maximally flexed forward and the forehead supported on folded arms which are resting on a table. The C7-T1 interspace is identified by the first prominent vertebral spinous process, which is C7, and a skin wheal of local anesthetic is injected in the midline.

Technique

A winged epidural needle is introduced in the midline, angled 30° cephalad and advanced using the hanging drop technique. When the needle is stabilized in the supraspinous ligament, the stylet is removed and a drop of local anesthetic is injected into the needle hub until it bulges outward enough to form a light reflection. The needle is then advanced slowly forward while keeping the thumbs out of contact with

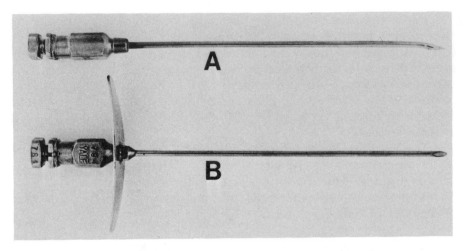

Figure 5-1. Epidural needles: **A** indicates the commonly used Tuohy needle with Huber point (Becton-Dickinson, New Jersey), and **B** the winged Tuohy, or Weiss, needle (Becton-Dickinson) flanged to facilitate control during use of the hanging drop technique.

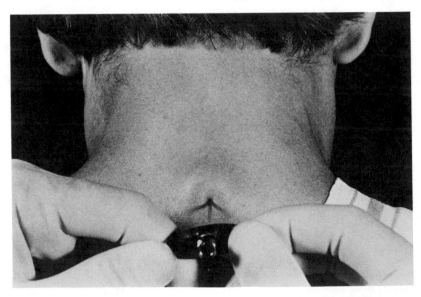

Figure 5-2. Cervical epidural block: Approach to the cervical epidural space. A winged Tuohy needle (Becton-Dickinson) allows precise control of the needle while keeping the thumbs out of contact with the hanging drop in the hub of the needle.

the drop (Fig. 5-2). If bone is encountered, the needle is redirected appropriately and walked off into the epidural space. Entry into the epidural space is evidenced by the hanging drop disappearing into the needle lumen as the negative pressure in the epidural space pulls it inward. Correct position of the tip may be confirmed by injecting local anesthetic or saline with a glass syringe and noting absence of resistance to injection. Another useful sign is the obvious variation in epidural pressure with respiration shown when another drop is placed in the hub. A deep inspiration will usually pull the drop into the needle. It should be noted that the depth from the skin to the epidural space and the cephalad angle vary widely between patients. The dose needed for a surgical anesthetic level for neck surgery is 6–8 ml of local anesthetic of a sensory blocking concentration.

Complications

The distance from the ligamentum flavum to the dura in the cervical region is 2 mm and from the dura to the spinal cord an additional 1–2 mm. Great care must be exercised, therefore, in maintaining absolute control of the needle in its passage into the epidural space to avoid cord injury or subarachnoid block. Motor concentrations of drugs must be avoided to prevent paralysis of the phrenic nerves.

THORACIC EPIDURAL BLOCK

This procedure allows a small anesthetic dose to provide anesthesia of the thoracic dermatomes and selectively block these areas while sparing the lumbar and sacral dermatomes. Thoracic epidural block is most valuable for postoperative pain relief permitting early ambulation after abdominal surgery.

Landmarks

The patient is placed in the sitting position with spine maximally flexed and leaning against a firm support. The interspace to be entered is identified. The T10-12 interspaces are easiest to approach (as explained in Anatomy, above). The back is prepped and a skin wheal is placed just lateral to the spinous process at the inferior aspect of the desired interspace (Fig. 5-3).

Technique

Through the above-marked wheal, a winged epidural needle is directed 10° medially and about 45° cephalad and inserted a few centimeters until stabilized by the tissues. The stylet is withdrawn and a

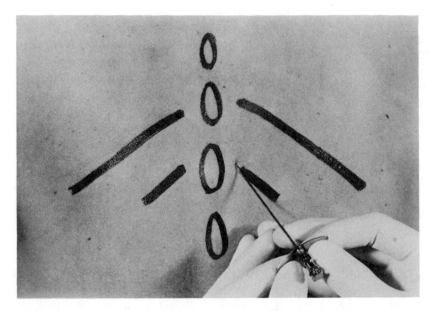

Figure 5-3. Thoracic epidural block: Approach to the thoracic epidural space. The needle is inserted just lateral to the spinous process at the inferior aspects of the interspace and directed 10° medially and 45° cephalad from the plane of the skin. Upon entering the interspinous ligament, the stylet is removed and a drop of saline or local anesthetic is placed in the needle hub. The needle is then advanced until lamina is contacted and then walked off the lamina in a cephalad direction to enter the epidural space. On entering the space, the hanging drop is suddenly aspirated into the needle by the negative intrapleural pressure.

drop of anesthetic solution placed in the needle hub. The needle is advanced into the epidural space using the hanging drop technique (see Cervical Epidural Blocks, above), which takes advantage of the negative pressure which exists in the thoracic epidural space. If bone is encountered, the needle is redirected cephalad and medial until it can be walked into the epidural space. The sitting position increases this negative pressure, increasing its reliability.

Entry into the epidural space should be checked by attaching a syringe with a test dose of local anesthetic to the needle hub. After negative aspiration for CSF or blood, the local anesthetic is injected. There should be no resistance to injection, and if the test dose fails to produce tachycardia or subarachnoid block, the anesthetic dose is injected. Because of the lesser capacity of the thoracic epidural space, the total dose of local anesthetic should be two-thirds of that which would be used in the lumbar epidural space.

Complications

The major complications are accidental dural puncture or intra-vascular injection. With too lateral a paramedian approach, pleural puncture is possible. The narrow epidural space in the thoracic region necessitates careful needle advancement to prevent injury to the spinal cord.

LUMBAR EPIDURAL BLOCK

As previously noted, the surgical indications for this block are similar to those for spinal anesthesia. The major differences are that epidurals take longer to set up and postdural puncture headache is avoided. Epidural blockade, therefore, is preferable in younger patients.

Landmarks

These are the same as for subarachnoid block with the L2-3, 3-4, and 4-5 interspaces most preferred.

Most Common Technique (Loss of Resistance)

Midline Approach

The selected interspace is palpated and a skin wheal is injected. If surgery on the knee, lower leg, or sacral dermatomes is to be performed, the L5-S1 interspace may be preferred so that a larger concentration of local anesthetic is introduced as close to the large L5 and S1 nerve roots (which are most difficult to anesthetize) as possible. The patient may be in the lateral or sitting position with the back maximally flexed. The lateral position usually is most comfortable for the patient. The positioning and skin preparation are as described for subarachnoid block. A 3.5-inch, 17- or 18-gauge Tuohy needle is directed toward the midline parallel with the sagittal plane and 10° cephalad and inserted 1–2 cm into the supraspinous ligament with the bevel (indicated by the notch in the hub) cephalad (Fig. 5-4). A 5 ml glass syringe should be lubricated with local anesthetic solution. One to two ml of local anesthetic and 1–2 ml of air are drawn into the syringe. The stylet is removed from the needle and the syringe is connected. The needle is advanced slowly while the thumb of the right hand maintains compression of the syringe plunger with a continuous in-and-out ballotting movement insuring that the plunger remains freely mobile. The fingers of the left hand grasp the needle, or the hub, with the back of the hand securely placed against the patient's back (Fig. 5-5) as the needle is slowly advanced.

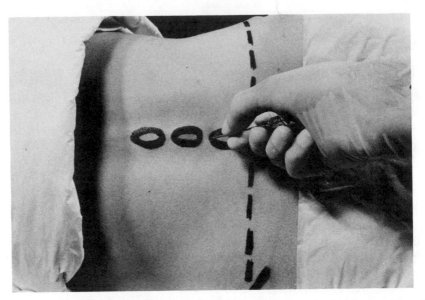

Figure 5-4. Lumbar epidural block: Midline approach to the lumbar epidural space. The needle entry point is in the midline of the interspace (L3-4 shown here) and is directed 10° cephalad until impinged in the interspinous ligament when the stylet is removed and the syringe attached.

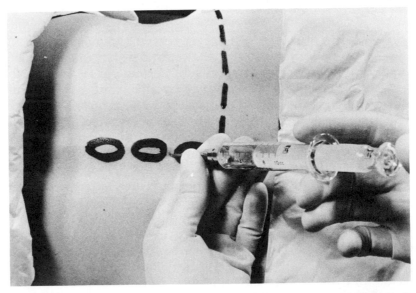

Figure 5-5. Lumbar epidural block: Technique for advancing needle into the epidural space. The fingers of the left hand grasp and slowly advance the needle while the back of the hand rests securely against the patient's back. The right hand balances the syringe while the right thumb maintains constant pressure on, or continuously ballotts, the plunger.

The key to recognition of the epidural space is the feel associated with changes in resistance to needle advancement coupled with the ease of local anesthetic injection. The spongy intraspinous ligament provides little resistance to needle penetration and the local anesthetic can be injected with little force on the plunger. Upon entering the ligamentum flavum, however, greater force is required to advance the needle and injection of local anesthetic through the needle becomes difficult.

The ligamentum flavum is several mm thick. As the needle passes beyond the ligamentum flavum into the epidural space, a sudden loss of resistance can be felt such that the plunger can be pushed in with almost no effort. The syringe is removed and the hub of the needle observed for blood or CSF. If none is seen, a test dose of local anesthetic is injected, and after a 30-second wait to rule out an intravascular injection, the remainder of the dose is injected slowly through the needle with repeated aspiration after each 5 ml injection.

If a catheter is to be used, it should be coiled and grasped in the little finger of the left hand. If a stylet is present in the catheter, it should be withdrawn 2–3 cm from the catheter tip. The catheter is then inserted through the needle with the bevel directed cephalad. The catheter is then advanced 2–3 cm beyond the tip of the needle. The distance from the needle hub to the skin is measured, most easily by measuring against the physician's hand (Fig. 5-6a) and the needle is removed a few mm at a time while the catheter is held immobile a few mm from the hub. When the needle is removed from the skin, the catheter is securely held with the hand braced against the patient's back while the needle is removed over the tail end of the catheter. The hand is placed against the patient's back (Fig. 5-6b) and the previous position of the needle hub before removal of the needle is reapproximated so that it may be determined if the catheter has moved during needle removal. The injection port is then attached to the tail of the catheter and a small syringe is connected. The catheter is then aspirated for CSF or blood, and if negative, 0.5 ml of local anesthetic is injected to insure that the catheter is patent. A pad is placed at the catheter entry site (Fig. 5-7) and the catheter is securely taped in place. The catheter injection port is taped in a secure, accessible place and the patient is positioned for surgery while the physician's hand is placed over the catheter entry site to prevent dislodgement during repositioning. If the surgical site is not to be in the midline, then the patient may be placed with the side to be operated on dependent until the block sets up. The effect of gravity on the establishment of blockade is less pronounced with epidural than with spinal anesthesia.

The blood pressure is checked every 30 seconds for the first 2 minutes, at which time a sensory exam is performed to rule out an accidental subarachnoid block. Thereafter, the blood pressure should be checked at least every minute until the block is stable, more often if

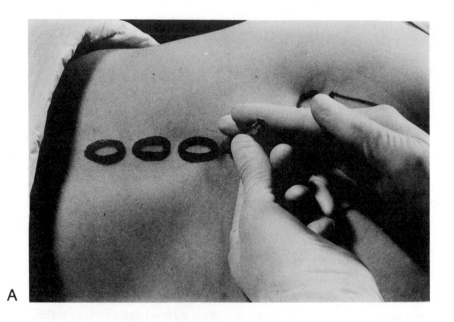

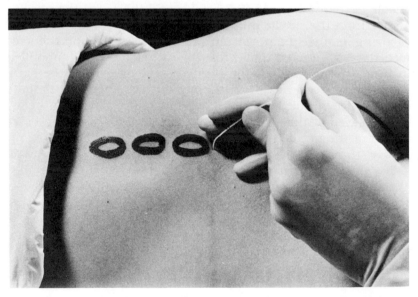

Figure 5-6. Lumbar epidural block: **(A)** The length of the catheter in the epidural space is exactly determined by measuring the distance from needle hub to skin against the physician's hand. Then **(B),** after threading the catheter into the epidural space, the needle is removed and the hand is placed in the same position on the patient's back, which allows approximation of the needle hub position. The catheter markings may then be compared to determine if the catheter changed position during needle removal.

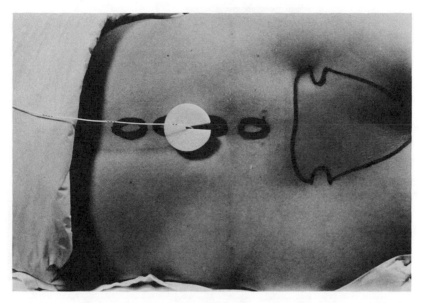

Figure 5-7. Lumbar epidural block: Padding the catheter entry site. A self-adhering foam pad or folded gauze sponge is placed at the site of catheter emergence and the catheter is taped over it to prevent kinking at the skin.

any change in blood pressure occurs. Sensory level should be checked every 5 minutes until a stable level is achieved and the highest level recorded on the anesthetic record for future reference. It should be remembered that the epidural catheter must be tested by an appropriate test dose before its position can be assumed to be safely in the epidural space.

Paramedian Approach

The advantages of this approach are that the spinous processes and interspinous ligament are avoided by the laterally placed needle. Therefore, the ability to enter the interlaminar space is not as dependent upon the patient's ability to flex his back. Also, the calcified supraspinous ligaments found in older patients, which can be difficult to penetrate, are avoided. The needle entry point is one thumb breadth lateral from the midline of the interspace (Fig. 5-8). If the patient is on the side, the entry point should be made on the dependent (or down) side for greatest success. The needle is aimed 10° cephalad and 20° medially. If bone is encountered, it is usually lamina. The needle is redirected medially and cephalad and walked off the bone, directly into the ligamentum flavum. The remainder of the procedure is identical to the midline approach.

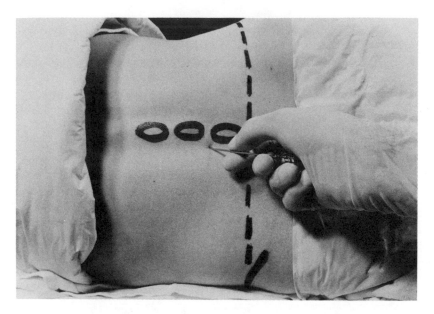

Figure 5-8. Lumbar epidural block—Paramedial Approach: The needle is inserted one thumb breadth lateral from the midline and aimed 10° cephalad and 20° medially into the interspinous ligament. After the stylet is removed and syringe attached, the needle is advanced into the epidural space utilizing the loss of resistance technique.

Common Problems in Lumbar Epidural Block

1. *Blood appears in the hub.* The needle should be repositioned at a higher interspace.
2. *CSF appears in the hub (dural puncture).* If surgery is to be performed, then the procedure should be converted to a subarachnoid anesthetic (See Chapter 4, Subarachnoid Block). After the appropriate dose of local anesthetic is injected, the needle is flushed with 0.25 ml of solution to insure that all the proper dose is instilled into the subarachnoid space rather than lying in the dead space of the large needle lumen. If the epidural is to be used for long-term pain relief, as in obstetrical labor, then attempted placement at a higher interspace may be performed as long as only small doses of local anesthetics are injected slowly (*only* through the catheter) and the patient checked frequently for possible high spinal blockade. It is not uncommon for epidurally injected local anesthetic to enter the subarachnoid space through a dural puncture at another level and cause a high spinal block. The patient should be observed for the develop-

ment of a postspinal headache. (See Section VI, Complications.)

3. *Catheter will not thread past needle tip.* Rotation of the needle 20° to each side or then 180° may allow passage. If not, then advancement of the needle 1–2 mm further into the epidural space may help. If a catheter without a stylet was first used, then one with a stylet (which is stiffer) should be tried. If a large volume of local anesthetic was not injected prior to threading the catheter because a high block level was not desired, then injecting 20 ml of preservative-free normal saline through the needle may distend the epidural space and allow passage of the catheter. If all else fails, and a catheter is required, placement at another interspace is recommended. Note: Once passed beyond the needle tip, the catheter should *never* be pulled back since it may be sheared off by the sharp bevel of the needle.

4. *Catheter enters a vein.* This is most common in pregnant patients since the epidural veins are enlarged. Blood may be aspirated or the test dose injected through the catheter may yield symptoms and signs of systemic local anesthetic toxicity indicating an intravenous bolus. (See Section VI, Complications.) The catheter may be withdrawn 1–1.5 cm and flushed with 0.5 ml of local anesthetic and then retested for intravenous placement. If retesting is negative, then further injections should be made slowly and cautiously while the patient is monitored closely for symptoms of systemic local anesthetic toxicity. If withdrawing the catheter does not bring the catheter tip out of the vein, then trying at another, usually more cephalad, interspace is recommended.

5. *Catheter enters subarachnoid space.* If anesthesia for a surgical procedure is required, then a continuous spinal technique (see Chapter 4, Subarachnoid Block) should be performed. If long-term pain relief is needed, the procedure described above for dural puncture should be followed.

6. *Inadequate block (level too low or block too weak).* One-half of the volume originally injected may be reinjected 20 min after the first injection. A solution of 2% lidocaine with epinephrine should be used since this provides the most profound block with the shortest onset time.

7. *Missed segments.* If the missed segments are unilateral, then the patient should be rolled on the side with the missed segments dependent. The catheter should be reinjected with an appropriate volume of 2% lidocaine with epinephrine. If this fails, then the catheter may be pulled back 1–2 cm, as the tip may be lodged in a root sleeve or in the lateral epidural space, and redosed. If the S1 or other sacral segment are missed bilat-

erally, then sitting the patient up and injecting 2% lidocaine with epinephrine may prove effective. If this fails, then a supplementary caudal block with 10–15 ml of 2% lidocaine with epinephrine will most often prove successful.

LOCAL ANESTHETICS FOR EPIDURAL BLOCK

Test Dose

The following local anesthetic solutions (3 ml) containing epinephrine, 1:200,000, will result in tachycardia and moderate rise in blood pressure within 45 seconds after intravascular injection, and will provide a safe but obvious level of spinal anesthesia when injected into the subarachnoid space.

Lidocaine	1.5–2%
Bupivacaine	0.5%
2-Chloroprocaine	3%

If epinephrine is not used, then 5 ml of the above local anesthetics will give symptoms of local anesthetic toxicity when injected as an intravascular bolus. If the entire dose is injected into the subarachnoid space, however, the level of spinal blockade may be higher than desired.

Caution should be exercised when bupivacaine is injected as a test dose. Unlike the other local anesthetics, bupivacaine does not always produce the classic symptoms associated with intravascular injection (sedation, circumoral numbness, tinnitus, etc.). Instead, patients may develop such nondescript complaints as headache, malaise or tremulousness. Epinephrine should be included in the test dose, therefore, to reliably rule out intravascular injection, particularly when higher concentrations of bupivacaine are to be used.

Dosage

Dosage depends on many factors, but approximate volumes of the above anesthetic solutions recommended for a 30-year-old patient of normal stature are as follows:

Level	T 10	T 4
Volume (ml)	20	30

These doses should be reduced by one third in pregnant women at term and for patients over 60 years of age. Patients suffering from severe atherosclerosis will require only about half of these volumes to achieve the same effect.

For abdominal surgery, lidocaine 1.5–2%, bupivacaine 0.5–0.75%, and 2-chloroprocaine 2–3% are generally used. The lesser concentrations will suffice for the lower abdomen but the higher concentrations are essential for upper abdominal procedures. Top-up doses are one-third of the initial dose and are usually administered when the block level begins to recede or when the patient notices the onset of discomfort. Alternatively, a top-up dose can be given by the clock, usually at 1–1.5-hour intervals for lidocaine, 1.5–2.5 for bupivacaine, and .75–1 for 2-chloroprocaine.

Probably the most difficult anesthesia to achieve is for surgery on the knee or posterior leg which is innervated by the most heavily myelinated nerve roots, L5 and S1. Block of these roots is best accomplished by insertion of the epidural needle at the lumbosacral interspace and the use of higher concentrations of local anesthetics (2% lidocaine, 0.5–0.75% bupivacaine). The patient should then be maintained in the lateral decubitus position with the leg to be operated dependent.

CONTRAINDICATIONS

These are the same as for subarachnoid block and include severe blood loss or shock, infection at the proposed site of needle entry, septicemia, and patient refusal. Progressive neurologic disease is a relative contraindication, and each case must be evaluated individually.

COMPLICATIONS

Complications of epidural analgesia resolve themselves into those due to technical difficulties, those due to systemic absorption of local anesthetics, and those resulting in neurological deficit. Massive subarachnoid injection secondary to accidental dural puncture results in high or total spinal block. Prompt ventilation and correction of hypotension can avoid permanent sequelae of anoxia. Several case reports have appeared in the literature describing permanent neurological deficits related to accidental total spinal block. All local anesthetics would appear to be implicated and it has been suggested that, should the total dose of drug be introduced into the subarachnoid space, an equal volume of spinal fluid be withdrawn. Evidence is lacking that such action will reduce the incidence of permanent neurological complications. Broken segments of epidural catheters may be left in situ unless they impinge on nerve roots, producing radiculopathy. Broken epidural needles should be removed surgically as soon as feasible. Systemic and neurologic complications are discussed in Section VI, Complications.

EPIDURAL BLOCK FOR OBSTETRICS

For labor and delivery, a segmental block from T10-L2 is necessary for pain relief during the early stages of labor. This is usually accomplished by placing an epidural catheter at the L2-3 intraspace and using 4–8 ml of 0.25% bupivacaine. Segmental analgesia is maintained by top-up doses as necessary. As the fetal head descends and presses against the floor of the pelvis, the sacral nerve roots may be blocked by administering larger doses of local anesthetic with the patient in a semisitting position. If complete perineal anesthesia is desired for delivery, a 10–15 ml dose of 1% plain lidocaine can be administered with the patient in the semisitting position enroute to the delivery room.

There are several concerns when epidural anesthesia is administered to a pregnant patient. To prevent slowing labor, the initial dose of local anesthetic should not be given until the cervix of the primiparous patient is 4–5 cm dilated, or 5–6 cm in the multiparous patient. Hypotension will also slow labor and can be partially prevented by the administration of 500 ml of balanced salt solution prior to the block and avoidance of the supine position with its associated aortocaval compression, as long as the epidural is being utilized. This is aided by a pillow or blanket placed under the patient's hip to keep the patient in the semilateral position.

EPIDURAL BLOCK FOR CESAREAN SECTION

The patient is given 1–1.5 liters of balanced salt solution intravenously before placement of the epidural needle. The usual total volume of local anesthetic administered is 20–23 ml, which will generally provide a T4 sensory level of anesthesia. A wedge should be placed under the patient's right hip to provide left uterine displacement to prevent aortocaval compression. Supplemental oxygen should be administered to the mother until the umbilical cord is clamped. Nausea and discomfort may occur, particularly if the uterus is delivered onto the abdomen during surgical repair. Supplemental narcotics and antiemetics are useful in this situation.

CAUDAL BLOCK

This block provides anesthesia of the perineum (lower sacral segments). The induction of epidural anesthesia involving *all* of the sacral or lumbar nerves or both can be accomplished by way of the sacral hiatus, which is the opening at the distal end of the sacral body, since the lumbar and sacral epidural spaces are contiguous. It is most commonly used for procedures in the perianal areas, such as hemorrhoidectomy. It can be used in children to provide reliable analgesia.

Landmarks

With the patient in the prone position with a pillow under the hips, or with the patient in the lateral Sim's position, the coccyx is identified with the palpating finger and the finger moved up to the first deep depression which can be noted on the sacrum. This is the sacral hiatus which provides entry to the caudal canal. On either side of the sacral hiatus, protuberances may be palpated. These are the sacral cornua which, with the sacral hiatus, form an inverted U (Fig. 5-9), although anomalies in this region are frequent. The caudal canal and sacral epidural space are protected from the overlying skin by the sacrococcygeal ligament, which must be perforated in order to produce caudal anesthesia.

Technique

The sacral hiatus is marked with a marking pencil and a skin wheal is made just below the arch of the U-shaped depression. A 3.5-inch, 22- or 20-gauge spinal needle with stylet in place is inserted perpendicular

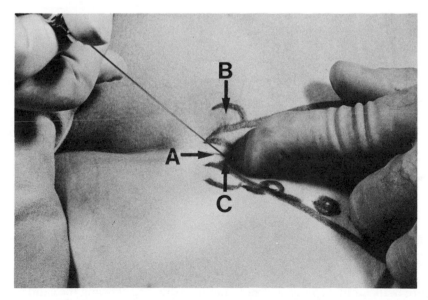

Figure 5-9. Caudal epidural block: **A** indicates the inverted U of the sacral hiatus, **B** the sacral cornua, and **C** the point of needle entry for caudal block.

to all planes of the skin through the cutaneous wheal until the "pop" of the sacrococcygeal ligament is felt. The needle is then rotated so that the bevel is ventral and the hub dropped so that the needle shaft is approximately 20°–30° in relation to the plane of the sacrum. A finger is placed over the upper portion of the hiatus to make certain that the needle does not ride on top of the sacrum. The needle is then advanced into the caudal canal approximately 2 cm (Fig. 5-10). The depth of the needle insertion may be checked by withdrawing the stylet and placing it alongside the needle to determine the location of the point (Fig. 5-11). After aspiration, a small quantity (3–5 ml) of saline should be injected while the opposite hand palpates over the dorsum of the sacrum. If the needle is riding superficial to the sacrum, the bolus of fluid will be felt with the palpating fingers. If the point of the needle is impinged in periosteum on the ventral surface of the sacrum, the solution can only be introduced with difficulty or not at all. Care must be taken in placement of the needle to make certain that the venous plexus on the ventral surface of the sacrum is not penetrated. A test dose of 3 ml of local anesthetic with 1:200,000 epinephrine should be injected to ascertain that neither a blood vessel nor the dural sac has been entered. Careful aspiration intermittently throughout injection is essential to avoid intravascular introduction of local anesthetics.

While the volume of the sacral canal is only 8–12 ml, local anesthetics injected into the caudal epidural space tend to leak through the

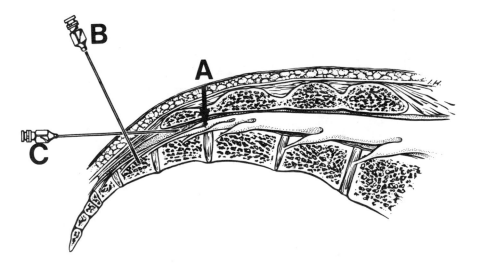

Figure 5-10. Caudal epidural block: Anatomic drawing showing the caudal canal **(A)**, the first position for entry of the needle **(B)**, and the needle within the canal **(C)**.

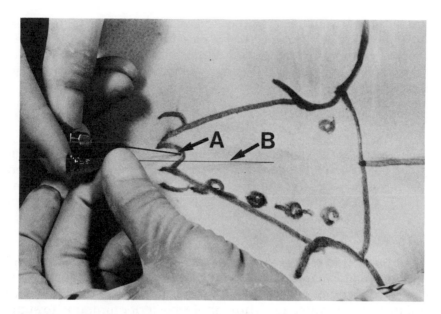

Figure 5-11. Caudal epidural block: Measuring depth of needle in caudal canal. **A** represents the needle in the caudal canal. The depth to which the needle is inserted is determined by placing the stylet **B** alongside the needle.

sacral foramina so that, in the nonparturient patient, up to 25 ml of local anesthetic may be required to produce adequate caudal anesthesia. Injection should be incremental to avoid an excessively high block. For prolonged surgery, a larger gauge epidural needle should be used and an epidural catheter inserted.

In children, the dose of local anesthetic solution to provide an L2 level of anesthesia is 0.5 ml/kg of lean body weight (0.7 ml/kg for a T10 level). Care must be taken that the dural sac is not entered since it extends further down into the sacrum than in the adult. Accordingly, a 1.5-inch, 22-gauge needle should be advanced just into the caudal canal and a test dose injected. Since this technique is usually performed on children under light general anesthesia, epinephrine should be included in the test dose to identify an accidental intravascular injection.

Complications

Because of the high incidence of posterior sacral defects in normal subjects, the most common complication of caudal block is failure to produce anesthesia. The local anesthetic may be deposited superficial to the sacrum when defects are present. Infrequently, the needle may be introduced through the sacrococcygeal ligament ventral to the sacrum. This would lead to injection of local anesthetic into the bladder, uterus, or retroperitoneal tissues. While such complications may not be of great significance in the nongravid patient, fetal absorption will be high and severe fetal toxicity may result during labor.

TRANSSACRAL BLOCK

The transsacral approach to the epidural space permits blocking of the individual sacral nerve roots or the entire contents of the sacral canal. It may be used for minor perianal procedures (S 5) or for management of the painful bladder. (See Section IV, Pain Blocks.)

Anatomy

The sacrum is made up of two layers of bone between which there is highly vascular and fatty tissue, a continuation of the lumbar epidural space. As such, it contains the posterior primary divisions of the sacral nerve roots which exit through the posterior foramina to supply the buttock area. The anterior primary divisions exit through the ventral foramina to supply innervation to the perineum and portions of the lower extremity. The superficial location of the posterior foramina lends itself to blockade of the sacral nerves.

Landmarks

With the patient in the prone position on a pillow placed under the hips, the posterior iliac spines, the most prominent protuberances of the sacrum, are palpated with the flat of the hand and marked. The two posterior superior iliac spines should form an equilateral triangle, with the apex being the sacral hiatus. A point is marked 1.5 cm medial and 1.5 cm cephalad to the posterior superior iliac spine to identify the first sacral foramen. A line is drawn from this point to the lateral surface of the sacral cornua on the same side. Two cm below the first sacral foramen on this line will be found the second sacral foramen, and subsequent foramina are an equal distance from the preceding foramen (Fig. 5-12).

Technique

A 3.5-inch, 22-gauge spinal needle with stylet in place is introduced through wheals placed at the above designated points. The needle is introduced perpendicular to all planes of the skin until the rim of the sacral foramen is contacted. At this point, a rubber marker is moved 1.5 cm along the shaft of the needle from the skin surface (Fig. 5-13).

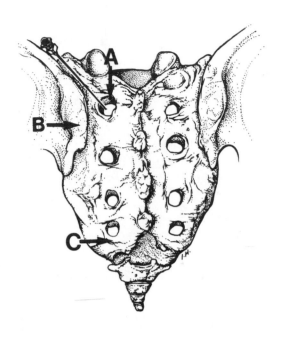

Figure 5-12. Transsacral nerve block: Anatomic drawing of the sacrum. The first sacral foramen **A** is located 1.5 cm medial and cephalad to the posterior superior iliac spine **B**. Subsequent foramina are located 2–2.5 cm caudad from the previous foramen on a line drawn from the first sacral foramen to the lateral aspect of the sacral cornua **C**.

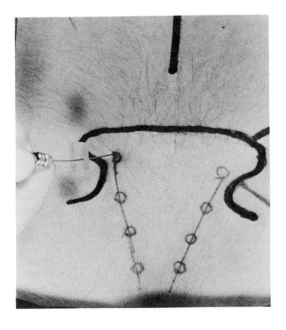

Figure 5-13. Transsacral nerve block: The needle is inserted perpendicular to all skin planes until the dorsal surface of the sacrum is contacted at the lateral superior edge of the sacral foramen. A rubber marker is then set at 1.5 cm from the skin surface.

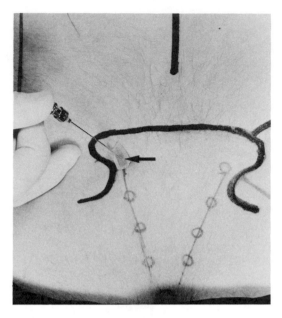

Figure 5-14. Transsacral nerve block: The arrow depicts the 45° medial and 45° caudad insertion of the needle to the depth of the rubber marker. After negative aspiration, local anesthetic can then be injected.

The needle is then slightly withdrawn and angled 45° caudad and 45° medial to drop into the sacral foramen to the depth of the marker (Fig. 5-14). A single sacral nerve root can be blocked with 1.5–2 ml of local anesthetic, and total caudal anesthesia may be obtained by the introduction through a single sacral foramen of a total volume of 15–25 ml of local anesthetic.

Complications

The most significant complication of transsacral nerve block, particularly at the S1 and S2 levels, is penetration of the dural sac. Injection of local anesthetic into the sac will produce subarachnoid block. In some instances, the dural sac may end at the level of the S3 foramen. Also, the large venous plexus on the ventral surface of the sacral space requires special care that intravascular injection does not occur. Penetration of the needle through the ventral foramina of the sacrum may perforate the rectum, uterus or bladder. ■

Section III

Peripheral Blocks

6

Head and Neck Blocks

TRIGEMINAL NERVE BLOCK

Blockade of the trigeminal nerve and its branches is used to provide localized anesthesia of the face for dental surgery and the management of facial pain.

Anatomy

The trigeminal nerve conveys sensation from the superficial and deep structures of the face and motor function to the muscles of mastication. The sensory and motor roots arise from the lateral part of the anterior surface of the pons and proceed forward in the posterior fossa of the skull to enter the middle fossa beneath the attachment of the tentorium cerebelli to the upper border of the petrous portion of the temporal bone.

In the middle fossa, the sensory root expands into the plexiform trigeminal ganglion. From this ganglion arise three large nerves—the first division or ophthalmic, the second or maxillary, and the third or mandibular. The motor nerve is incorporated entirely within the mandibular division.

The *ophthalmic nerve* passes toward the orbit in the middle fossa of the skull and at the superior orbital fissure separates into the lacrimal, frontal and nasociliary divisions. The lacrimal division passes between the contents of the orbit and the periosteum to the anterior portion of the orbit and supplies the lacrimal gland, the conjunctiva and the lateral portion of the eyelid.

The frontal nerve passes through the superior orbital fissure and courses above the ocular muscles, where it divides into two branches. The larger branch, the supraorbital nerve, leaves the orbit through the supraorbital foramen to supply the forehead and scalp to the vertex, the frontal sinus, and the upper eyelid. The other branch, the supratrochlear nerve, courses forward to reach the medial portion of the supraorbital margin, where it leaves the orbit to supply the skin of the medial forehead and upper eyelid.

The *maxillary nerve* leaves the ganglion and, after passing through the foramen rotundum, crosses the pterygopalatine fossa to enter the infraorbital fissure. It exits on the face through the infraorbital foramen. In the pterygopalatine fossa, the nerve gives off branches to the soft and hard palate and the mucous membrane of the inferior concha of the nasal cavity.

The infraorbital nerve gives off the anterior superior alveolar nerve supplying branches to the incisor, canine, premolar and first molar teeth. On the face, it supplies the skin and conjunctiva of the lower lid, the skin of the side of the nose, and the cheek and upper lip.

The *mandibular nerve* exits the skull through the foramen ovale, where the large afferent and smaller efferent root form a single trunk with anterior and posterior divisions. The anterior, or motor, division supplies the muscles of mastication. The posterior division divides into the lingual and inferior alveolar nerves.

The lingual nerve passes medial to the lateral pterygoid muscle and then between the medial pterygoid and the mandible. In the mouth, it lies beneath the mucous membrane about 1 cm below and behind the last molar. It supplies sensation to the anterior two-thirds of the tongue and the mucous membrane of the floor of the mouth.

The inferior alveolar nerve passes under the lateral pterygoid muscle to reach the ramus of the mandible and enters the mandibular canal through the mandibular foramen. It supplies sensation to the lower teeth. It terminates by dividing into a mental and incisor branches. The mental branch exits onto the face through the mental foramen and supplies the skin of the chin and lower lip. The incisor branch supplies the canine and incisor teeth.

GASSERIAN GANGLION BLOCK

Landmarks

A skin wheal is raised on the cheek 3 cm lateral to the angle of the mouth at the level of the second molar tooth. The midpoint of the zygomatic arch on the same side should be marked as well at a point 2 cm posterior to this point (Fig. 6-1).

Technique

A 3.5-inch, 22-gauge needle is introduced through the skin wheal and directed superior and posteromedial so that the point is directed, in the lateral plane, toward the mark at the midpoint of the zygomatic arch and, in the frontal plane, directly toward the pupil. When bone is contacted at the infratemporal plate in the pterygoid fossa just anterior to the foramen, the needle is then withdrawn and redirected toward the mark 2 cm posterior to the midpoint of the zygomatic arch to enter Meckel's cave (Fig. 6-2). As soon as paresthesias to the lower jaw are obtained, injection of 3–5 ml of local anesthetic will block all divisions of the nerve. An alternate technique is to use the first needle insertion as a guide for a second needle directed toward the foramen. This allows for determination of needle depth and direction.

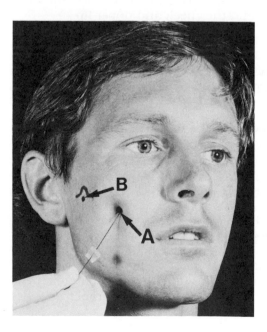

Figure 6-1. Gasserian ganglion block: A 22-gauge needle is inserted at point **A**, 3 cm lateral to the angle of the mouth at the level of the second molar tooth, and directed superior and posteriomedial so that the point is directed, in the lateral plane, toward the mark at the midpoint of the zygomatic arch **B** and, in the frontal plane, directly toward the pupil. When bone is contacted in the pterygoid fossa just anterior to the foramen, the needle is then withdrawn and redirected toward the mark at the midpoint of the zygomatic arch to enter Meckel's cave.

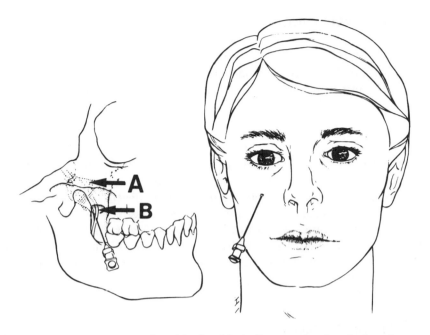

Figure 6-2. Gasserian ganglion block—Meckel's cave: Anatomic drawing showing **(A)** the Gasserian ganglion in the pterygoid fossa (Meckel's cave); and **(B)** the mandibular branches of the trigeminal nerve.

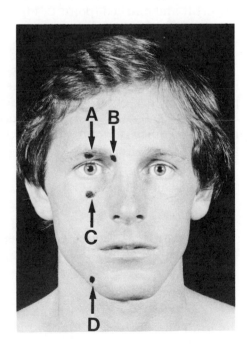

Figure 6-3. Trigeminal nerve block—superficial branches: **A** is the location of the exit onto the face of the supraorbital nerve, **B** the supratrochlear nerve, **C** the infraorbital nerve, and **D** the mental nerve. Note that **A**, **C**, and **D** are in the same sagittal plane.

OPHTHALMIC NERVE BLOCK

Landmarks

The supraorbital notch is palpated at the upper rim of the orbit 2.5 cm from the midline. A skin wheal is raised at this point (point A, Fig. 6-3).

Technique

A 1-inch, 25-gauge needle is inserted through the skin wheal and directed in a posterior and cephalad direction to contact the rim of the supraorbital notch. At this point, 3 ml of local anesthetic are deposited outside of the supraorbital foramen. Unless a neurolytic block is contemplated, the foramen need not be entered (Fig. 6-4). The supratrochlear nerve is blocked by introducing 2 ml of local anesthetic at the junction of the medial border of the upper rim of the orbit with the root of the nose (point B, Fig. 6-4).

MAXILLARY NERVE BLOCK

Landmarks

The infraorbital foramen is palpated 1 cm below the inferior rim of the orbit and marked (point C, Fig. 6-4).

Technique

A skin wheal is raised at the above point and a 23-gauge 1.5-inch needle is inserted through the wheal to contact the foramen. When paresthesias are obtained, 3 ml of local anesthetic is deposited at the foramen (Fig. 6-4). As in the supraorbital block, the foramen need not be entered unless a neurolytic procedure is contemplated.

MANDIBULAR NERVE BLOCK

Landmarks

The patient is requested to open the mouth as wide as possible. The point midway on the zygomatic arch is marked (Fig. 6-5).

Technique

A 3.5-inch, 22-gauge needle is inserted through a wheal raised at the midpoint of the zygomatic arch into the space formed by the arch

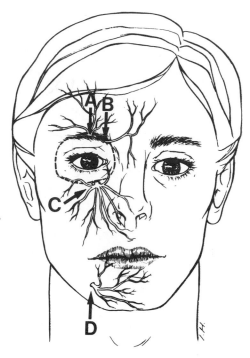

Figure 6-4. Trigeminal nerve block: Anatomic drawing of cutaneous branches of the trigeminal nerve. **A** represents the supraorbital, **B** the supratrochlear, **C** the infraorbital, and **D** the mental nerves exiting their respective foramina. (Reproduced from Carron H: Control of pain in the head and neck. Otolaryngol Clin North Am 14(3), August 1981. With permission.)

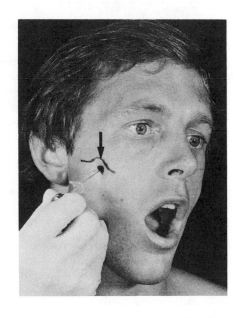

Figure 6-5. Mandibular nerve block—external approach: With the patient's mouth wide open, a 7–8 cm needle is inserted into the space formed by the zygomatic arch (arrow) and the incisura mandibula and anterior to the condyle of the mandible. The needle is advanced perpendicular to all planes of the skin to the base of the infratemporal fossa where paresthesias are sought before injection of local anesthetic.

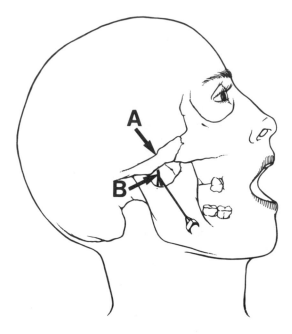

Figure 6-6. Mandibular nerve block: Anatomic drawing showing the relationship of the zygomatic arch **A** to the incisura mandibula **B** anterior to the condyle of the mandible. (Reproduced from Carron H: Control of pain in the head and neck. Otolaryngol Clin North Am 14(3), August 1981. With permission.)

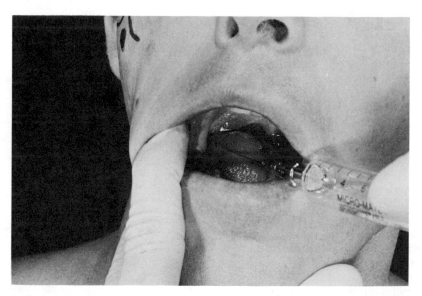

Figure 6-7. Mandibular nerve block—intraoral approach: The dental and lingual branches are blocked where the nerve enters the mandibular canal approximately 1 cm posterior and inferior to the last molar tooth of the lower jaw. The ridge of the opening of the canal can be palpated. Local anesthetic is deposited to the lingual side of the canal to provide anesthesia of the lower teeth and posterior two-thirds of the tongue.

and the incisura mandibula anterior to the condyle of the mandible. The needle is advanced perpendicular to all planes of the skin to the base of the infratemporal fossa. When paresthesias are obtained, 3 ml of local anesthetic are injected (Fig. 6-6).

The dental and lingual branches may be blocked intraorally where the nerve enters the mandibular canal approximately 1 cm posterior and inferior to the last molar tooth of the lower jaw. The ridge of the opening of the canal can be palpated. Three ml of local anesthetic deposited to the lingual side of the canal will provide anesthesia of the lower teeth and posterior two-thirds of the tongue (Fig. 6-7). ■

7

Intercostal Block

Intercostal block is used to provide anesthesia of the thorax and abdominal wall and in the management of rib fractures. When it is used in combination with sympathetic blocks that provide visceral anesthesia, various diagnostic and therapeutic thoracic and abdominal procedures may be performed.

Anatomy

The intercostal nerves derive from the primary rami of T1–T12. Some fibers from T1 join with the C8 nerve root to become the lowest trunk of the brachial plexus while the 12th nerve combines with the first lumbar to become the ilioinguinal and iliohypogastric nerves. The intercostal nerves run segmentally under the respective ribs. As each emerges from its intervertebral foramen in the paravertebral space, it is separated from the pleura by the endothoracic fascia. At the costal angle, the nerve passes along the caudal margin of the rib and continues below the artery and vein in the costal groove where it lies between the internal and external intercostal muscles. In the midaxillary line, each intercostal nerve gives off a lateral cutaneous branch, and near the sternum, an anterior cutaneous branch that innervates a narrow band of skin on the ventral and lateral aspects of the thorax or abdomen.

Techniques

The patient is preferably placed in a lateral position with the arm drawn forward and upward over the head to expose the region of the costal angles. With the patient in this position, the lower margin of the ribs can easily be palpated, facilitating the block. As the fingers palpate the lower margin of the rib at its angle, the overlying skin is drawn cephalad (Fig. 7-1). A 1.5-inch, 22-gauge short beveled needle is inserted toward the rib in a slightly cephalad direction until contact is made with bone. The needle is then walked caudad on the rib until it slips off the inferior margin. The overlying skin is now released and the needle is then advanced approximately 2–3 mm under the margin of the rib and 3–5 ml of local anesthetic are injected (Fig. 7-2). The number of ribs to be injected depends upon the area of surgical incision, although if the abdomen is to be opened the lower 6–8 intercostals must be blocked. Figure 7-3 depicts the cross-sectional anatomy of intercostal block.

PARAVERTEBRAL APPROACH

Landmarks

The major bony landmarks for paravertebral thoracic block are the spinous and transverse processes of the vertebrae. The patient is placed in the prone or lateral position. The spinous processes are marked, as are points 3 cm lateral to the spinous processes. The thoracic spinous processes are long and angled caudad. Therefore, in the upper thoracic area, the spinous process will be palpated opposite the transverse process of the vertebra below. In the midthoracic area, the overlap may be as much as two vertebrae (Fig. 7-4).

Technique

Skin wheals are raised over the marked sites opposite the spinous processes. A 3.5 in., 22-gauge spinal needle is introduced slowly through each wheal perpendicular to all planes of the skin until the transverse process is contacted. A needle marker is set at 2.5 cm from the skin and the needle is then withdrawn to the subcutaneous tissue. It is reinserted 30° medial and caudad up to 2.5 cm to contact the postero-lateral body of the vertebra just under the transverse process, where 3–5 ml of local anesthetic are deposited. If bone is not contacted by the

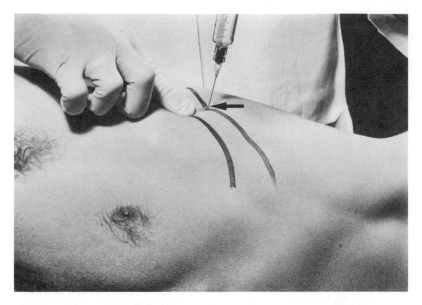

Figure 7-1. Intercostal nerve block—step 1: The arrow indicates the skin pulled up over the rib to be blocked with the needle probing for the inferior rib margin.

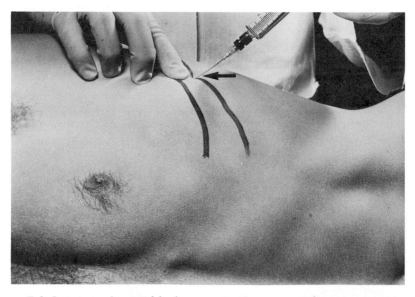

Figure 7-2. Intercostal nerve block—step 2: The arrow indicates insertion of the needle 2–3 mm under the inferior rib margin after skin retraction is released. Note direction of needle insertion.

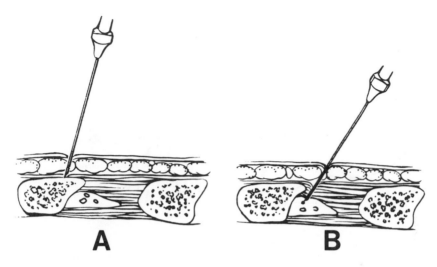

Figure 7-3. Intercostal nerve block: Anatomic drawing showing **(A)** step 1, and **(B)** step 2.

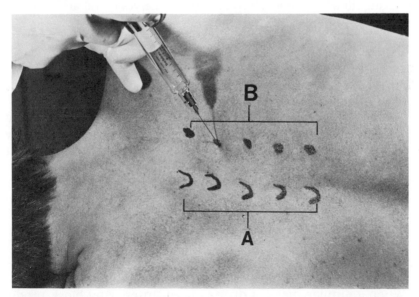

Figure 7-4. Intercostal nerve block—paravertebral approach: **A** indicates the tips of the spinous processes and **B** the site of insertion of needles 3 cm lateral to the spinous processes. Needles should be directed 45° medially and 30° caudad to pass just under the transverse processes where the local anesthetic is injected.

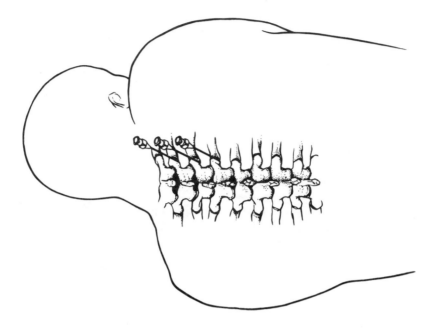

Figure 7-5. Intercostal nerve block—paravertebral approach: Anatomic drawing showing relationship of intercostal nerves to thoracic spinal transverse processes.

2.5 cm depth, the needle is withdrawn and directed more medially. Anatomical relationships are shown in Figure 7-5.

There is considerable cutaneous overlap of the intercostal nerves, and therefore, one level above and below the desired dermatomal levels should be blocked. If abdominal surgery is to be performed, the intercostal block should be supplemented with subcutaneous infiltration along the lateral border of the rectus, and local anesthetic should be deposited in the posterior rectus sheath to block the perforators innervating the rectus abdominis muscle.

COMPLICATIONS

When a similar mass of drug is used, intercostal block produces significantly higher blood levels of local anesthetic than brachial or epidural block or local infiltration. Blood levels frequently reach convulsive thresholds when several ribs are blocked (See Section VI, Complications). If intercostal block is performed paravertebrally, the long root sleeves of the intercostal nerves may be entered, resulting in subarachnoid block. The pleura may also be penetrated since the intercostal nerves lie in close proximity to the parietal pleura. ■

8

Abdominal Blocks

OBTURATOR NERVE BLOCK

Obturator nerve block may be used in combination with femoral and sciatic block to provide anesthesia of the leg. It may also be used to provide anesthesia of the hip for manipulations or pain control.

Anatomy

The obturator nerve is the major anterior derivative of the lumbar plexus, being comprised of the ventral roots from L2, L3, and L4 (Fig. 8-1). The nerve is formed in the psoas major muscle and emerges from the medial border of that muscle at the approximate level of the sacro-iliac joint and with the external iliac vessels anterior to it. It enters the pelvis, coursing in a caudal and ventral direction to run along the lateral wall of the pelvis to the obturator canal, through which the obturator vessels and the obturator nerve enter the thigh. Usually, the nerve divides into its anterior and posterior branches when located in the obturator canal, although this division may occur during its intrapelvic course.

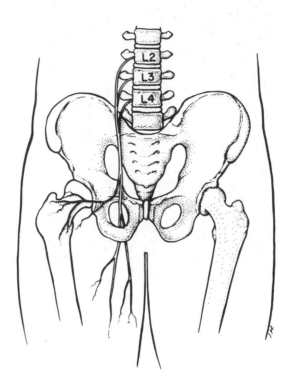

Figure 8-1. Obturator nerve: Anatomic drawing of origin of the obturator nerve from the ventral roots of L2, L3, and L4 showing its peripheral distribution to the hip joint, the adductor muscles, and a cutaneous area of the medial thigh.

Before, or as the nerve enters the thigh, a branch may be given to the anteromedial portion of the hip joint. The anterior branch innervates the anterior set of adductor muscles and a variable cutaneous area of the medial thigh. The posterior branch pierces the obturator externus muscle and descends on the adductor magnus muscle to innervate the deep adductor muscles of the thigh, and terminally, sends a branch to the articular surface of the knee.

Landmarks

The patient is placed supine and the public tubercle on the side to be blocked is palpated. A mark that is 1–2 cm lateral and 1–2 cm caudad to this tubercle is placed on the skin. (Fig. 8-2).

Technique

A 3.5-inch, 22-gauge needle is inserted perpendicular to all planes of the skin until the mediosuperior border of the public bone is contacted. The needle is then withdrawn and the tip is directed slightly lateral and inferior to bypass the pubic bone and pass into the obturator

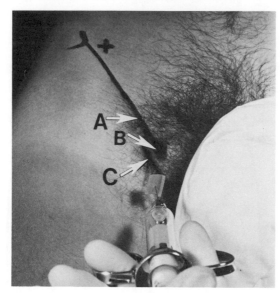

Figure 8-2. Obturator nerve block: **A** represents the inguinal ligament, **B** the pubic tubercle, and **C** the initial site of injection for the obturator nerve. After the needle contacts the superior lateral margin of the obturator foramen, a marker is set 1.5 cm from the skin surface. The needle is then withdrawn and reintroduced slightly medial and inferior to bypass the pubic bone and pass into the obturator canal to a depth of approximately 2–3 cm.

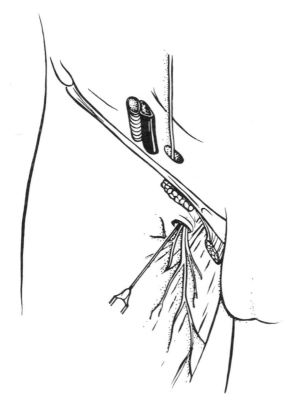

Figure 8-3. Obturator nerve block: Anatomic drawing of obturator nerve block, showing relationship of needle to obturator foramen and obturator nerve.

canal to a depth of approximately 2–3 cm past the previous bony contact. The needle is aspirated to identify if the vessels that accompany the nerve have been entered. If the aspiration is negative for blood, 10–15 ml of local anesthetic solution are injected. Some authors recommend an injection of an additional 10 ml of local anesthetic solution as the needle is withdrawn (Fig. 8-3).

Complications

Complications of obturator nerve block relate to improper needle placement with possible visceral puncture or intravascular injection. Local anesthetic block of the obturator nerve may produce temporary instability of the lower extremity due to paralysis of the adductor muscles of the thigh.

ILIOINGUINAL, ILIOHYPOGASTRIC, AND GENITOFEMORAL BLOCKS

These blocks may be used together in conjunction with local infiltration of the line of incision to provide anesthesia for procedures involving the inguinal area, i.e., herniorrhaphy, orchiectomy, node biopsy, or vas deferens ligation.

Anatomy

The lumbar plexus is formed in the psoas major muscle from the anterior roots of spinal nerves L1-4. There frequently is a T12 component and occasionaly one from L5. The *iliohypogastric nerve* is a derivative from T12 and L1 that courses in a ventral and caudad direction between the transversus abdominis muscle (transversalis muscle) and the internal oblique muscle after piercing the transversalis muscle at a point just medial to the anterior superior iliac spine (ASIS). It passes 2–3 cm medial to the ASIS and provides sensation to the skin overlying the lateral buttock, the inguinal ligament, and some innervation to the superficial muscles of the lower abdominal wall. There are frequently anastomotic connections between the iliohypogastric and the lower intercostal nerves, so that the cutaneous distribution is not necessarily strictly dermatomal.

The *ilioinguinal nerve* is an L1 derivative originating slightly below the iliohypogastric nerve but paralleling its course. It, too, emerges through the transversus abdominis muscle behind the iliac crest, but soon thereafter courses anteriorly and caudally between the internal and external oblique muscles. It provides sensation to the skin over the superficial inguinal ring, the scrotum or labia, and the adjacent thigh. The iliohypogastric and the ilioinguinal nerves run in an anteromedial direction after passing the ASIS and become superficial, with terminations in cutaneous branches to the skin and in branches to the inguinal canal, where they lie anterior to the cord.

The *genitofemoral nerve* originates from the L1 and L2 roots of the lumbar plexus. It courses over the anterior surface of the psoas major muscle and behind the peritoneum. The nerve usually divides just above the inguinal ligament. The genital branch crosses the external iliac artery and enters the inguinal canal through the internal inguinal ring. It lies posterior to the spermatic cord and innervates the cremaster muscle. It exits by the external inguinal ring to provide sensation to the skin of the scrotum or labia major. The femoral branch courses laterally to the external iliac vessels and under the inguinal ligament to provide sensation to the skin of the upper femoral triangle.

Landmarks

The ASIS must be located. The point of infiltration for blockade of the iliohypogastric and ilioinguinal nerves will be 2.5–3 cm medial and 2–3 cm caudal to the ASIS (Fig. 8-4). Successful blockade will result if local anesthetic is placed between the appropriate muscle layers of the anterior abdominal wall. The genitofemoral nerve can be approached by a lower abdominal injection that requires identifying the pubic tubercle (Fig. 8-4).

Technique

A skin wheal is made at the point of entry of the needle for the iliohypogastric and ilioinguinal block. The first infiltration of about 10 ml of local anesthetic solution is made after a 1.5–3.5-inch, 22-gauge needle (depending upon the size of the patient) is placed perpendicular to the skin and directed laterally until it contacts the inner surface of the iliac bone. The infiltration is performed while the needle is withdrawn. Once the needle is back to the subcutaneous level, it is directed in the dorsal direction but more medially than before to pierce the external oblique, internal oblique, and transversalis fascia. Five to 7 ml of local anesthetic solution are injected as the resistance of each of the three fascial layers is passed (Fig. 8-5).

For genitofemoral block, from the pubic tubercle, a fanlike infiltration of the muscle layers in a lateral, cranial, and medial fashion with 5–7 ml of local anesthetic solution in each direction is made (Fig. 8-5).

Figure 8-4. Ilioinguinal, iliohypogastric, and genitofemoral nerve blocks: **A** represents the anterior superior iliac spine and **B** the inguinal ligament. **C** is the point of injection for the ilioinguinal and iliohypogastric nerves 2.5–3 cm medial and 2–3 cm caudad to the anterior superior iliac spine. **D** is the site of injection for the genitofemoral nerve just distal and lateral to the pubic tubercle. Injection should be carried out in a fan-like manner penetrating the superficial fascia.

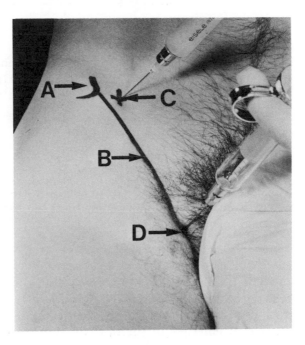

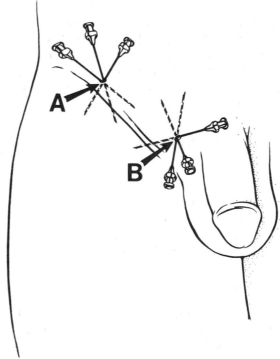

Figure 8-5. Ilioinguinal, iliohypogastric, and genitofemoral nerve blocks: Anatomic drawing showing the technique of injecting in a fan-like manner to block all superficial branches of the ilioinguinal and iliohypogastric nerves **(A)** and the genitofemoral nerve **(B)**.

Complications

The major complication of this combination of ilioinguinal, ilio-hypogastric and genitofemoral block is peritoneal puncture. In this highly vascular area, hematoma formation is common, but of little lasting consequence.

PUDENDAL NERVE BLOCK

Pudendal nerve block provides anesthesia of the perineum and pelvic floor. It is most commonly used in obstetrics for episiotomy and perineal repair.

Anatomy

The pudendal nerve is derived from the second, third, and fourth branches of the sacral plexus. It leaves the pelvis by passing through the lower portion of the greater sciatic foramen and under the piriformis muscle. It emerges in the buttock area by passing between the lower border of the piriformis muscle and the upper border of the superior gemellus muscle. After coursing over the gemellus muscle and passing behind and laterally to the ischial spine and sacrospinous ligament, it returns to the pelvis heading toward the perineum via the lesser sciatic foramen. It traverses the lateral wall of the ischiorectal fossa to lie medial to the obturator internus muscle in the pudendal canal. Here it gives off the inferior rectal nerves. Thereafter, it divides into its perineal and dorsal penile (or dorsal nerve of the clitoris) branches to innervate the skin of the external genitalia.

Transvaginal Approach

Landmarks

The patient is placed in the lithotomy position and the ischial spine and the sacrospinous ligament are palpated through the vagina (Fig. 8-6). One must be sure that the ischial spine (which is more posterior) is located and not the more anterior ischial tuberosity.

Technique

A needle guide should be used, and if so, it is placed in the vagina with the tip on the mucosa overlying the junction of the ischial spine and the sacrospinous ligament that attaches there. A 3.5-inch, 22-gauge needle is introduced through the vaginal mucosa and a "pop"

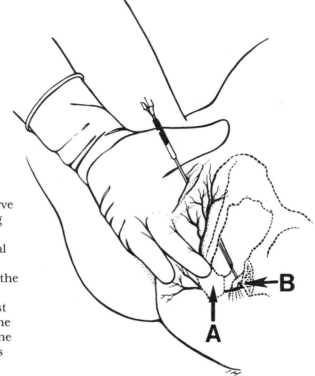

Figure 8-6. Pudendal nerve block: Anatomic drawing showing transvaginal approach to the pudendal nerves. **A** indicates the ischial tuberosity and **B** the ischial spine. Injection should be carried out just medial to point **B** after the "pop" of penetration of the sacrospinous ligament is felt.

will be felt as it penetrates the sacrospinous ligament. After aspiration is negative for blood, 10 ml of 1% lidocaine solution is injected. This technique is then repeated on the other side for bilateral block.

Some authors note that this technique has a higher success rate than the transperineal approach because of its relative simplicity and the fact that it is less painful for the patient. Its advantages seem to be the use of less local anesthetic, the shorter distance of needle penetration, and the decreased incidence of complications such as hematoma of the perineum and rectal puncture.

Perineal Approach

Landmarks

The lithotomy position is used. The ischial tuberosities are marked, and the ischial spine is palpated. It may be helpful to have the middle finger in the rectum to identify rectal puncture.

Technique

Skin wheals are placed at a point that is 2–3 cm posterior and medial to the ischial tuberosity (Fig. 8-7). A 3.5-inch, 22-gauge needle is inserted through the wheal to contact the bony prominence of the ischial tuberosity. Then 5–10 ml of local anesthetic solution are injected laterally and under the tuberosity to anesthetize the inferior pudendal nerve. The needle is moved to the medial side of the tuberosity where another 10 ml are injected.

Then the needle is advanced carefully another 2–3 cm, using the finger in the rectum as a guide (and as a detector of rectal perforation), whereupon approximately 10 ml of local anesthetic are injected. This should place local anesthetic in the ischiorectal fossa, which is roughly bounded by the ischial spine and ischial tuberosity.

Finally, with the index finger in the vagina as a guide, the needle is advanced in a dorsal lateral direction (posterior) to the ischial spine (which is posterior to the tuberosity) where the sacrospinous ligament

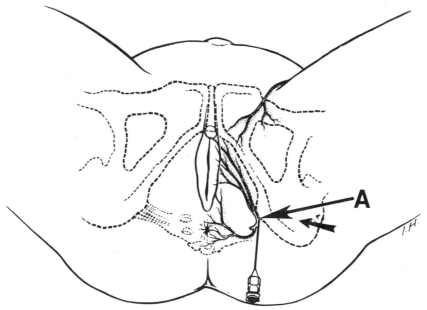

Figure 8-7. Pudendal nerve block—perineal approach: The arrow points to the ischial tuberosity. A finger in the rectum or vagina palpates for the ischial spine **(A)**. The needle is introduced posteromedial to the ischial tuberosity and directed medial and cephalad to meet the palpating finger. A "pop" is felt when the needle penetrates the sacrospinous ligament and local injection is made at this point.

can be penetrated. Once this has occurred (a distinct "pop" is usually felt) and aspiration of the needle is negative for blood, an additional 5– 10 ml of local anesthetic solution are injected. The entire procedure is then repeated on the other side.

The advantage of this approach is that the pudendal nerve and the posterior cutaneous nerve of the thigh (an S1, 2, 3, derivative which emerges through the greater sciatic foramen below the piriformis and medial to the sciatic nerve) which innervate the perianal area of the perineum and the lower labia are blocked. If this block is used for obstetrical anesthesia, subcutaneous infiltration 2–3 mm from and parallel to the labia major from the midpoint of the labia to the mons pubis is done to anesthetize the terminal branches of the iliohypogastric, ilioinguinal, and genitofemoral nerves.

Complications

Pudendal nerve block is usually employed during the second stage of delivery in the pregnant female. In this group of patients, vascularity of the pelvic organs is increased and the potential for rapid absorption of local anesthetic drug into the circulation is enhanced. Systemic toxic reactions may result. Also, improper needle placement, i.e. without a guiding finger in the vagina or rectum, may result in the drug being introduced into the fetal skull or the pelvic viscera.

PARACERVICAL BLOCK

This block provides anesthesia of the lower segment of the uterus and cervix. While rarely used for vaginal delivery, it provides excellent anesthesia for dilatation and curettage procedures.

Anatomy

Uterine pain is a sympathetically-mediated phenomenon. White rami communicantes fibers of the T11 and T12 spinal nerves allow sensory impulse transmission to the lower thoracic and lumbar sympathetic chain. Pain is transmitted from the uterus and the uterine plexus through the pelvic ganglia and pelvic sympathetic plexus to the hypogastric nerve and the superior hypogastric plexus. The superior hypogastric plexus sends impulses into the CNS through the T11 and T12 spinal nerve sympathetic connections. Paracervical block is performed at a level in the chain of sensory input where transmission via the pelvic sympathetic ganglia and plexus is interrupted.

Landmarks

The patient is placed in the lithotomy position and the lateral fornix of the vagina is located.

Technique

With the patient in the lithotomy position, the index and middle fingers of one hand are used to direct a needle guide into the lateral fornix of the vagina at the 3 o'clock position (Fig. 8-8). A needle is passed through the guide to contact the vaginal mucosal wall and then passed another 1.5 cm or so further into the uterosacral ligament. If aspiration of the needle is negative for blood, 10–15 ml of local anesthetic solution are injected. The procedure is repeated on the other side with the needle placed at the 9 o'clock position.

Usually 0.5–1% lidocaine without epinephrine is used and the block lasts 60–75 minutes. Bupivacaine 0.25% lasts about 90–100 minutes. The chief use of this block is for interruption of pregnancy or uterine biopsy in the poor-risk patient.

Complications

Paracervical block in the nonpregnant female is comparatively free of complications. While absorption of local anesthetic is fairly rapid, toxicity is rarely seen.

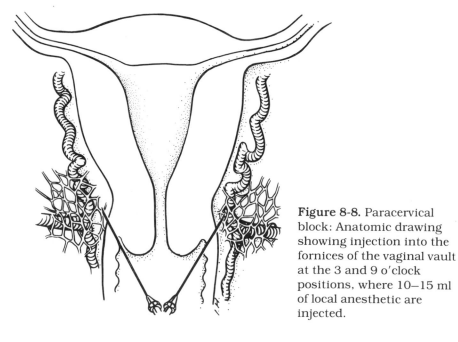

Figure 8-8. Paracervical block: Anatomic drawing showing injection into the fornices of the vaginal vault at the 3 and 9 o'clock positions, where 10–15 ml of local anesthetic are injected.

In the parturient patient, the greatest risk is to the fetus. Para-cervical block produces increased tone of the uterus with uterine vaso-constriction and decreased villous blood flow. Rapid absorption of local anesthetic into the maternal systemic circulation aand thence into the placental and fetal circulation, combined with uterine vasoconstric-tion, can be responsible for fetal bradycardia, acidosis and death. There are reports in the literature as well of injection of local anesthetic directly into the fetal skull, resulting in fetal mortality. The block is, therefore, preferably reserved for the poor risk, nonpregnant patient or for abor-tion in the first trimester.

PENILE BLOCK

Penile block provides surgical anesthesia of the penis and can be used for circumcision or relief of postsurgical pain in children.

Anatomy

The right and left dorsal nerves of the penis are derived from the pudendal nerve (a derivative of sacral roots 2, 3, and 4). The dorsal nerves enter the penis after passing underneath the symphysis pubis and penetrating the suspensory ligament of the penis. They run along the dorsal surface of the penis under the deep fascia (Buck's fascia), but are not as deep as the corpora cavernosa. A short distance after entering the penis, they begin providing multiple branches that run a circumferential pattern around the penis to provide sensation to the lateral and ventral aspects.

Landmarks

The patient is placed in a supine position and the lower border of the symphysis publis above the root of the penis is palpated. Marks are made at the 2 o'clock and 10 o'clock positions at the base of the penis (Fig. 8-9).

Technique

A 0.75-inch, 25-gauge needle is placed through the skin just to one side of the midline until the lower border of the symphysis pubis is contacted. The needle is withdrawn slightly and moved progressively in a caudal direction until bone is no longer contacted. A "pop" may be felt as the deep fascia of the penis is pierced (Fig. 8-10). Careful aspi-ration of the needle is performed to ascertain if the blood vessels that accompany the dorsal nerve have been entered. If so, the needle is repositioned until no more blood is aspirated. One must be careful not

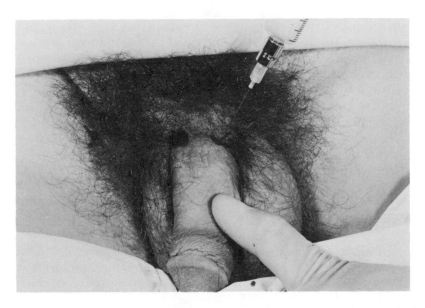

Figure 8-9. Penile block: A 25-gauge, .75-inch needle is inserted through the skin at the 2 and 10 o'clock positions at the base of the penis until the lower border of the symphysis pubis is contacted. The needle is withdrawn slightly and moved progressively in a caudad direction until bone is no longer contacted. A "pop" may be felt as the deep (Buck's) fascia of the penis is pierced. If aspiration is negative for blood, local anesthetic is injected.

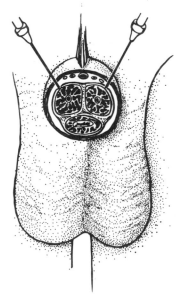

Figure 8-10. Penile block: Anatomic drawing showing injection of local anesthetic beneath Buck's fascia. Subcutaneous injection lateral to the penis on both sides may supplement injection of the penile nerves.

to replace the needle too superficially. When the aspiration is negative, 10 ml of the local anesthetic solution is injected. The procedure is repeated on the opposite side.

An injection performed too closely to the pubic bone will block the dorsal nerve before any significant branching has taken place. It is then possible that sensation may remain intact along the undersurface of the penis. This situation can be managed by a supplemental injection of local anesthetic solution along the lateral surface of the penis.

Complications

Hemorrhage into the shaft of the penis is the major complication of penile block. This is best avoided through use of fine caliber needles. It is recommended that local anesthetic solutions containing epinephrine not be used in performing this block, as the possibility of intense, prolonged vasoconstriction of the penile end-arteries could result in necrosis. One must also avoid the temptation to place a circumferential ring of local anesthetic around the base of the penis as this, too, could result in necrosis. ■

9

Upper Extremity Blocks

ELBOW BLOCK

Brachial plexus block can be supplemented with block of the median, radial, and ulnar nerves at the elbow; or, these blocks may suffice for anesthesia of the forearm and hand in the event that a tourniquet is not to be used.

Anatomy

The *ulnar nerve* in its course to the distal third of the upper arm perforates the medial muscular septum and enters the extensor compartment. It traverses the elbow and the ulnar nerve sulcus, which is situated on the posterior aspect of the medial epicondyle of the humerus.

The *median nerve* runs along the inner border of the upper arm in the large neurovascular sheath. At the elbow, in the antecubital fossa, the nerve lies medial to the brachial artery and is covered by the aponeurosis of the biceps muscle.

The *radial nerve*, after passing in the spiral groove around the posterior-lateral aspect of the humerus, continues in front of the elbow to lie in the groove between the brachioradialis and the biceps muscles. At the elbow, these anatomical locations lend themselves well to block of the major nerve trunks. Figure 9-1 shows the deep anatomy of the major nerves of the upper extremity at the elbow.

Landmarks

The ulnar nerve can be palpated in the sulcus of the medial condyle of the humerus when the arm is held in a flexed position. Pressure in the sulcus will produce paresthesias into the ring and little fingers. The median nerve is located on the ulnar side of the brachial artery just above the flexion crease of the elbow. Its location in the antecubital fossa is fairly superficial. The radial and lateral cutaneous nerves have as their landmark the radial border of the biceps tendon and the insertion of the brachioradialis muscle on the humerus. In this sulcus between these two muscles the lateral cutaneous nerve of the forearm is fairly superficial, while the radial nerve lies in close proximity to the humerus itself.

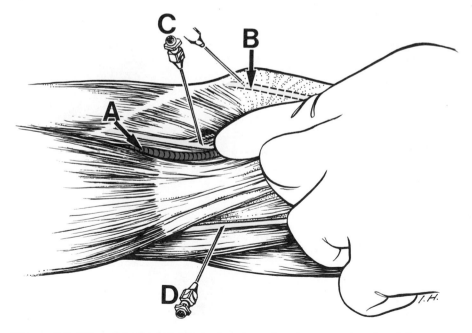

Figure 9-1. Elbow block: Anatomic drawing of major nerve trunks of the upper extremity at the elbow. **A** is the brachial artery, **B** the ulnar nerve, **C** the median nerve, and **D** the radial nerve.

Technique

The ulnar nerve is blocked by inserting a fine gauge needle parallel to the long axis of the arm and into the sulcus containing the ulnar nerve (Fig. 9-2). Paresthesias are usually obtained and a total volume of 5 ml of local anesthetic is adequate to block the nerve at this location.

To approach the median nerve, a 1.5-inch, 22-gauge needle is inserted just above the flexion crease of the elbow to the ulnar side of the brachial artery with the needle angled approximately 30° lateral and cephalad from the perpendicular. As the needle is advanced, paresthesias may be obtained at a depth of 1–2 cm, at which time 3–5 ml of local anesthetic should be injected (Fig. 9-3).

The radial nerve is blocked by inserting a needle just above the flexion crease of the elbow with the arm extended, between the biceps and the insertion of the brachioradialis. The needle should be directed approximately 30° medial and cephalad and advanced until it contacts the lateral condyle of the humerus. Then 5–7 ml of local anesthetic solution should be injected as the needle is slowly withdrawn from this location. When just subcutaneous, an additional 3–5 ml should be injected to block the lateral cutaneous nerve of the upper forearm (Fig. 9-4).

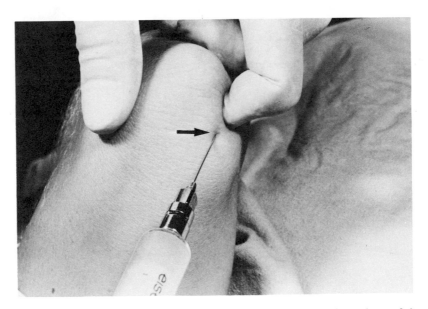

Figure 9-2. Elbow block—ulnar nerve: The arrow indicates the sulcus of the medial condyle of the humerus containing the ulnar nerve. The needle should be inserted into the sulcus in the long axis of the humerus.

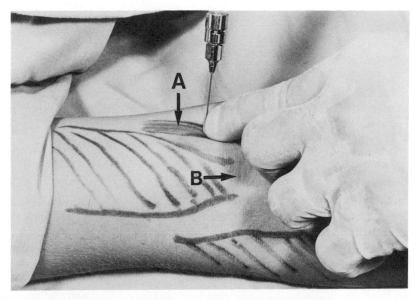

Figure 9-3. Elbow block—median nerve: The needle is inserted just medial to both the brachial artery **A** and the biceps tendon **B** and directed 30° medial to contact the medial condyle of the humerus just above the flexion crease of the elbow. Five ml of local anesthetic are injected.

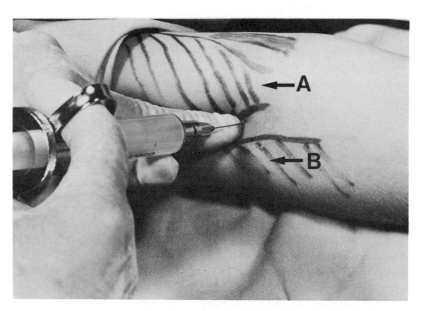

Figure 9-4. Elbow block—radial nerve: **A** represents the biceps tendon and **B** the brachioradialis muscle. The needle is inserted between these two structures just above the flexion crease of the elbow and directed 30° medial until it contacts the lateral condyle of the humerus. Five ml of local anesthetic are injected as the needle is withdrawn.

WRIST BLOCK

Blockade of the ulnar, median, and radial nerves at the wrist provides anesthesia of the hand. These blocks are useful in supplementing brachial plexus block for hand surgery since the onset time for anesthesia is shortened and a high success rate is attained.

Anatomy

At the level of the proximal crease of the wrist, the median nerve lies superficially on the anterior aspect of the forerm immediately radial to the tendon of the palmaris longus, or between it and the tendon of the flexor carpi radialis. The median nerve innervates the palmar surface on the radial side of the hand to the midline of the ring finger.

The ulnar nerve at the wrist accompanies the ulnar artery, and about 5 cm proximal to the wrist divides into dorsal and palmar branches. The dorsal branch proceeds to reach the dorsal aspect of the wrist and the ulnar side of the dorsum of the hand. The deep branch of the nerve supplies sensation to the ulnar side of the palmar aspect of the hand, the little finger, and ulnar side of the ring finger, and motor function to the intrinsic muscles.

Approximately 5–7 cm proximal to the wrist, the radial nerve passes beneath the tendon of the brachioradialis and lies subcutaneously on the dorsal aspect of the forearm at the level of the wrist. Here it divides into several branches supplying the radial 3.5 fingers of the dorsum of the hand.

Technique

For block of the median nerve at the wrist, a 1-inch, 25-gauge needle is inserted between the tendons of the palmaris longus and flexor carpi radialis at the level of the proximal crease of the wrist (Fig. 9-5). The needle should be introduced perpendicular to all planes of the skin and 3–5 ml of local anesthetic injected as the needle is advanced toward the dorsal surface of the wrist.

The ulnar nerve is blocked by palpating the ulnar artery and introducing a needle between it and the flexor carpi ulnaris approximately 3 cm above the flexion crease of the wrist (Fig. 9-6). Bone should be contacted above the ulnar styloid process and 3–5 ml of local anesthetic injected on withdrawing the needle.

The radial nerve can be blocked approximately 7 cm above the wrist by infiltrating under the palmar border of the brachioradialis tendon (Fig. 9-7) and then injecting a subcutaneous wheal at this level running dorsally around the radial border of the wrist to the styloid process of

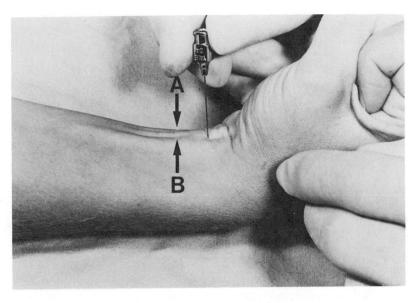

Figure 9-5. Wrist block—median nerve: The needle is inserted between the palmaris longus tendon **A** and the flexor carpi radialis tendon **B** at the proximal flexion crease of the wrist. Local anesthetic is injected as the needle is advanced toward the radius.

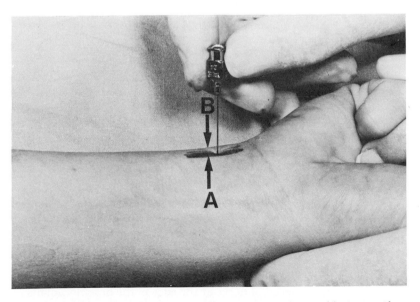

Figure 9-6. Wrist block—ulnar nerve: The needle is inserted between the ulnar artery **A** and the flexor carpi ulnaris tendon **B** and is directed toward the styloid process of the ulna.

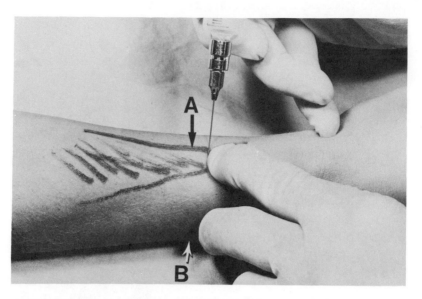

Figure 9-7. Wrist block—radial nerve: The needle is inserted under the ulnar border of the brachioradialis tendon **A** to block the radial nerve as it becomes superficial at this point. The block may be augmented by a subcutaneous bracelet of local anesthetic running from point **A** to point **B** on the dorsum of the wrist.

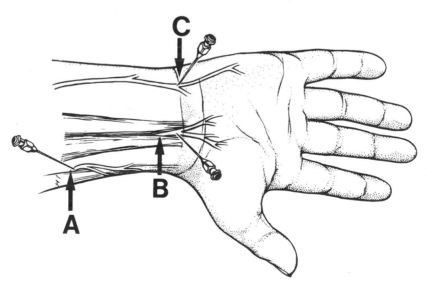

Figure 9-8. Wrist block: Anatomic drawing of relationships of major nerves at the wrist. **A** indicates the radial nerve at the edge of the brachioradialis tendon, **B** the median nerve between the palmaris longus and flexor carpi radialis tendons, and **C** the ulnar nerve between the ulnar artery and the tendon of the flexor carpi ulnaris.

the ulna. Figure 9-8 shows the anatomic relationships of the deep structures at the wrist. Figure 9-9 shows the cutaneous distribution of anesthesia produced by wrist block.

Complications

Elbow and wrist blocks are singularly devoid of complications. The volume of drug used is usually insufficient to produce a systemic reaction. Intraneural injection, particularly of the ulnar nerve at the elbow, can result in postblock neuritis, however. Seeking for paresthesias will enhance this possibility.

DIGITAL BLOCK

Digital nerve block of fingers and toes is easily accomplished by the injection of 0.5–1 ml of local anesthetic without epinephrine on either side of the base of the respective digit via a 25-gauge 1-inch needle (Fig. 9-10). The nerves lie in proximity to the palmar and the dorsal surfaces of the digits (Fig. 9-11).

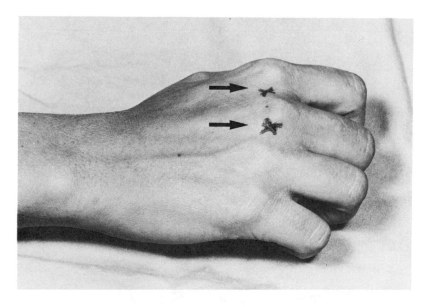

Figure 9-10. Digital nerve block: The arrows indicate the points of needle insertion opposite the heads of the metacarpals. Both dorsal and palmar branches are blocked by continuing injection during advancement of the needle toward the palm.

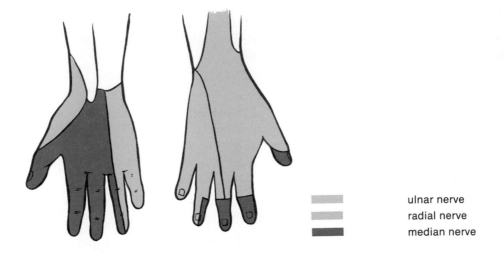

ulnar nerve
radial nerve
median nerve

Figure 9-9. Wrist block—cutaneous anesthesia: Cutaneous distribution of anesthesia with block of major nerves at the wrist.

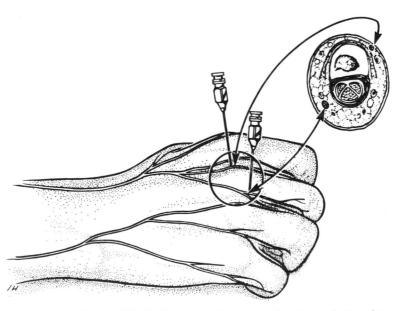

Figure 9-11. Digital nerve block: Anatomic drawing showing relationships of the digital nerves in the hand.

Complications

The greatest danger in performing digital nerve blocks is interference with blood supply through vascular compression or vasoconstriction. Vascular compression occurs when too large a volume of local anesthetic is used to block the digital nerves. This is particularly true when the block is performed on an already traumatized and edematous digit. Epinephrine should never be used with local anesthetics for digital block since resultant constriction of small end arteries may be prolonged and blood supply to the distal digit occluded. ■

10

Lower Extremity Blocks

All or part of the lower extremity can be anesthetized using a combination of nerve blocks when spinal and epidural blocks are not considered suitable for a particular patient. These regional blocks have a high success rate and few complications.

Anatomy

The nerves to the lower extremity originate in the lumbar and sacral plexuses. The lumbar plexus, consisting of nerve root components from L1 to L5, gives rise to the lateral femoral cutaneous, obturator and femoral nerves which provide sensory innervation to the lateral thigh and anteromedial aspect of the leg. The femoral nerve extends below the knee, becoming the saphenous nerve. The sacral plexus, consisting of L4 to S4 nerve root components, gives rise to the posterior femoral cutaneous and sciatic nerves which provide sensory innervation to the posterior and lateral aspect of the leg. The sciatic nerve extends below the knee, dividing to become the sural, posterior tibial, and peroneal nerves.

SCIATIC NERVE BLOCK

Posterior Approach

Landmarks

The patient may be placed prone or in the lateral position with the side to be blocked superior and the top leg in 45° of flexion. The posterior superior iliac spine and the superior aspect of the greater trochanter are marked, and a line is drawn joining the two. From the midpoint of this line, a perpendicular line is drawn in a caudad direction extending 4–5 cm (Fig. 10-1). This point is marked as the point of needle entry. An alternative means of finding the position of the needle entry is to draw another line from the greater trochanter to the sacro-coccygeal junction. The perpendicular line previously drawn is then extended down to where it intersects this line for the point of needle insertion (Fig. 10-2). The deep anatomic structures are shown in Figure 10-3.

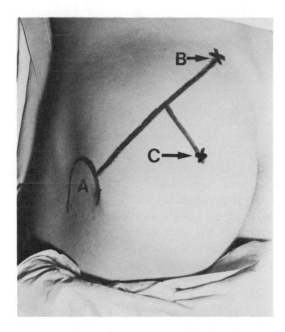

Figure 10-1. Sciatic nerve block—posterior approach: A line is drawn joining the superior aspect of the greater trochanter **A** and the posterior superior iliac spine **B**. From the midpoint of this line, another line is drawn perpendicular and caudad for 5 cm. Point **C** overlies the sciatic nerve.

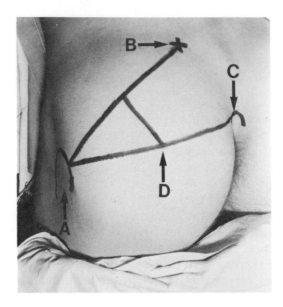

Figure 10-2. Sciatic nerve block—alternate posterior approach: **A** represents the superior border of the greater trochanter, **B** the posterior superior iliac spine, and **C** the sacral hiatus. Where the line drawn from the midpoint of the line **AB** intersects with line **AC** is the location of the greater sciatic notch **D**.

Technique

A 3.5-inch, 22-gauge spinal needle is inserted through a skin wheal perpendicular to all planes of the skin until it strikes the bony pelvis. This usually occurs at 2–5 inches in depth. When bone is encountered, the needle is walked in a caudad direction in the plane of the perpendicular line until the needle tip walks off of bone into the sciatic notch. If a paresthesia is not elicited, the needle should be fanned in the plane perpendicular to the course of the nerve until paresthesias are obtained. It should be noted that the paresthesia should extend below the knee to ensure that the nerve itself has been touched and not confused with referred pain from stimulation of the periosteum, which may radiate to the posterior thigh. When the appropriate paresthesia has been obtained, the needle fixed, and after negative aspiration in two planes, 20 ml of local anesthetic are injected. Since this is the largest nerve in the body, 20–30 minutes is usually required before surgical anesthesia can be obtained. The posterior femoral cutaneous nerve that lies in close proximity to the sciatic is usually blocked as well.

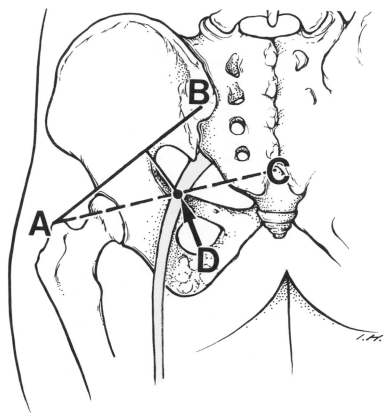

Figure 10-3. Sciatic nerve block—posterior approach: Anatomic drawing showing the relationship of the sciatic nerve to pelvic structures. **A** is the superior border of the greater trochanter, **B** the posterior superior iliac spine, **C** the sacral hiatus, and **D** the point of insertion for block of the sciatic nerve.

Lithotomy Approach

The lithotomy approach to the sciatic nerve offers the advantage of allowing the patient to remain supine. Anatomy is similar to that already described except that the nerve is blocked at a slightly more caudad point.

Landmarks

The patient is placed in the supine position. The leg to be blocked is flexed as much as possible and held in that position by an assistant.

The ischial tuberosity and the greater trochanter are marked and a straight line joining the two is drawn. The midpoint of this line is the point of needle entry (Fig. 10-4).

Technique

A 3.5-inch spinal needle is inserted perpendicular to all planes of the skin and advanced as before until paresthesias are obtained. In seeking a paresthesia, the needle should be fanned in the plane of the line that was drawn (perpendicular to the course of the nerve) until a paresthesia is obtained, and then local anesthetic is injected as described (Fig. 10-5).

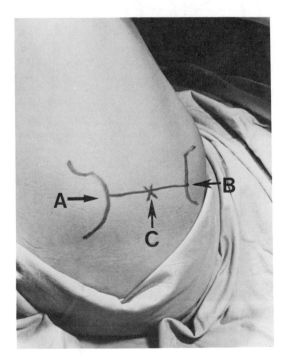

Figure 10-4. Sciatic nerve block—lithotomy approach: The leg to be blocked is flexed at the knee and hip and held by an assistant. A line is drawn from the superior border of the greater trochanter **A** to the lateral border of the ischial tuberosity **B**. The midpoint **C** of this line is the point of entry for sciatic nerve block.

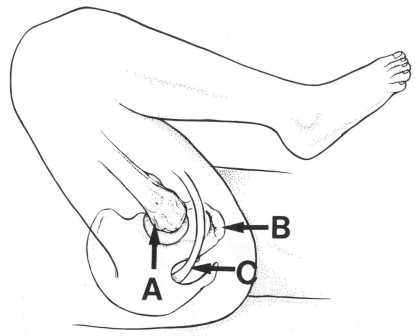

Figure 10-5. Sciatic nerve block—lithotomy approach: Anatomic drawing indicating greater trochanter **A**, lateral border of ischial tuberostiy **B**, and sciatic nerve **C**.

Complications

The only complications seen with sciatic nerve block are those resulting from intravascular injection of the local anesthetic or from damage to nerve fibers in seeking paresthesias. Systemic absorption of local ancsthctics from soft tissues of the lower extremity is slow and the drug rarely reaches significant blood levels. If paresthesias are obtained upon injection, the needle must be withdrawn slightly until injection is accomplished without discomfort.

FEMORAL NERVE BLOCK

Sciatic–Femoral Block

Combination sciatic–femoral nerve block is indicated for surgery below the knee without use of a tourniquet. The femoral nerve innervates the medial leg and is approached as described for the lumbar plexus block (see Section I, Chapter 3) except that only 20 ml of local anesthetic is injected. Although less local anesthetic is required than for the lumbar plexus block, large quantities are still used and caution against toxicity is advised. Figure 10-6 illustrates the areas of anesthesia produced by this combined block.

Complications

Because of the close proximity of the femoral nerve to the artery and vein at the femoral triangle, perforation of a vessel is not uncom-

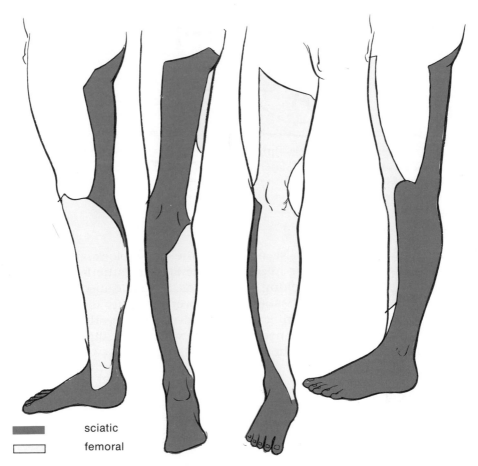

sciatic
femoral

Figure 10-6. Sciatic–femoral nerve block: Anatomic drawing showing the cutaneous distribution of anesthesia following sciatic-femoral nerve block.

mon. Hematoma formation may occur but is of little major significance. If the needle traverses the femoral sheath, pelvis viscera may be entered and damaged, although such complications have not been reported. Dysesthesias may follow intraneural injection or seeking for paresthesias.

COMMON PERONEAL BLOCK

The common peroneal nerve provides sensation to the lateral calf and foot.

Landmarks

The common peroneal nerve is readily accessible to block as it passes behind the head of the fibula. A point is marked just posterior to the inferior border of the head of the fibula (Fig. 10-7).

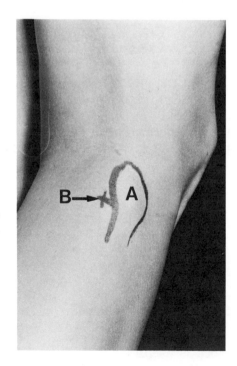

Figure 10-7. Common peroneal nerve block: **A** indicates the head of the fibula on the posterolateral aspect of the leg just below the knee joint. **B** indicates the point of injection of the common peroneal nerve just posterior and inferior to the head of the fibula. Injection is carried out in the long axis of the fibula to avoid injection into the nerve.

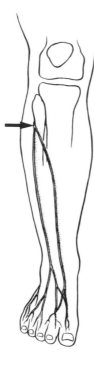

Figure 10-8. Common peroneal nerve block: Anatomic drawing showing relationship of the common peroneal nerve (arrow) to the head of the fibula.

Technique

A 1.5-inch, 22-gauge short bevel needle with syringe attached is introduced parallel and cephalad to the shaft of the femur from the above point until paresthesias into the foot are obtained. The needle is then withdrawn from the body of the nerve and 5–7 ml of local anesthetic is injected. Anatomical relations are depicted in Figure 10-8.

Complications

Complications relate only to dysesthesias secondary to intraneural injection.

SAPHENOUS BLOCK

Sciatic–Saphenous Block

Saphenous nerve block (at the knee) combined with sciatic nerve block is useful for procedures below the knee not requiring a tourniquet, since the saphenous nerve is the only component of the lumbar plexus and femoral nerve that provides sensory innervation to the medial leg below the knee.

Landmarks

The saphenous nerve is located in the subcutaneous tissue on the medial side of the knee below the knee joint. It is posteromedial to the large saphenous vein, which can often be identified (Fig. 10-9).

Technique

Subcutaneous infiltration on the medial aspect of the knee just below the joint with 10 ml of local anesthetic will provide anesthesia along the medial side of the lower leg to the ankle (Fig. 10-10). The sciatic nerve block will provide anesthesia to the rest of the lower leg.

Complications

When a saphenous block is performed in patients with varicose veins, there is increased risk of intravascular injection of local anesthetic. Dysesthesias may follow intraneural injection or seeking for paresthesias.

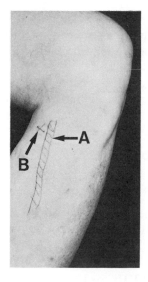

Figure 10-9. Saphenous nerve block: The saphenous vein **A** is located on the medial aspect of the leg just below the knee joint with the leg dependent. A needle is inserted at point **B** to infiltrate medial and deep to the saphenous vein to block the saphenous nerve.

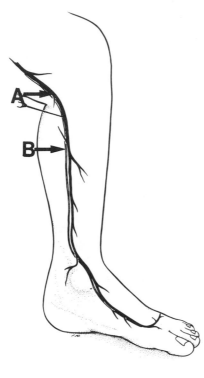

Figure 10-10. Saphenous nerve block: Anatomic drawing showing relationship of saphenous vein **A** to saphenous nerve **B**.

ANKLE BLOCK

This block is indicated for surgical procedures on the foot that do not require a tourniquet. It is particularly useful for forefoot amputations secondary to ischemic disease, since the block increases skin blood flow. With use of long-acting local anesthetics, excellent postoperative analgesia is possible. Epinephrine should not be used in patients with ischemic lesions of the foot. This block is performed in two phases: on the anterior aspect of the ankle, and then on the posterior aspect.

Anterior Aspect

Landmarks

The patient is placed supine with the foot and leg supported at midcalf by folded sheets. The surface landmarks are shown in Figure 10-11. Deep structures are shown in Figure 10-12. The nerves to be blocked on the anterior aspect are the deep peroneal, the saphenous, and superficial peroneal nerves. In surgical procedures involving the

Figure 10-11. Ankle block—anterior: The patient is requested to flex the great toe to identify the extensor hallucis longus and the tibialis anterior tendons. At the anterior ankle crease on a line joining the malleoli and between these tendons, point **A** indicates the site of needle insertion for the deep peroneal nerve. The saphenous nerve **B** is blocked by infiltrating around the saphenous vein just superior and anterior to the medial malleolus. Point **C** just superior and anterior to the lateral malleolus is the site for needle insertion to block the superficial peroneal nerve. Block may be enhanced with subcutaneous infiltration starting at the lateral malleolus and ending at the medial malleolus.

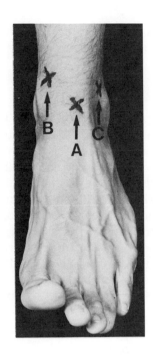

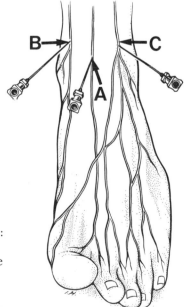

Figure 10-12. Ankle block—anterior: Anatomic drawing showing relationships and distribution of the deep peroneal nerve **A**, the saphenous nerve **B**, and the superficial peroneal nerve **C**.

lateral aspect of the foot, the deep peroneal block is omitted since this nerve provides sensory innervation to the great and second toes only.

Technique

The deep peroneal nerve is located by having the patient dorsiflex the foot and toes to identify the two large tendons of the extensor hallucis longus and tibialis anterior. Between these two tendons at the level of the superior aspect of the malleolus, a 22-gauge, 1.5-inch needle is inserted perpendicular to all planes of the skin until bone is felt. Seven ml of local anesthetic is injected in a fanwise manner in a mediolateral plane to infiltrate the entire compartment. The saphenous and superficial peroneal nerves are then blocked by means of subcutaneous infiltration along the anterior half of the ankle at the level of a line drawn between the upper portion of the medial and lateral malleoli. Special attention is given to deposition of local anesthetic just lateral to the greater saphenous vein, where the saphenous nerve lies. A total of 10 ml of local anesthetic is usually required.

Posterior Aspect

Landmarks

The posterior aspect of the foot is blocked using the landmarks shown in Figure 10-13, the deep anatomy of which is depicted in Figure 10-14. Anesthesia produced by combined anterior and posterior ankle block is shown in Figure 10-15.

Technique

With the patient in the lateral position, the posterior tibial nerve is blocked by introducing the needle just medial to the Achilles tendon at the level of the proximal aspect of the medial malleolus and directing it as if aiming at the second toe. If the posterior tibial artery can be palpated, then the needle is directed just medial to it and advanced until paresthesia or bone is encountered. If a paresthesia is obtained at this depth, 5 ml of local anesthetic are injected. If a paresthesia is not obtained, then the compartment is filled with a fanning technique in the mediolateral plane with a total of 10 ml of local anesthetic. The sural nerve is then blocked by placing the needle just lateral to the Achilles tendon at the level of the upper border of the lateral malleolus, and directed toward the little toe until bone is felt. Seven ml of local anesthetic are injected in a fanning technique in the mediolateral plane.

Figure 10-13. Ankle block—posterior: To block the tibial nerve **A**, a needle is inserted at the superior border of the medial malleolus between it and the Achilles tendon **B**, and directed toward the second toe. The sural nerve **C** is blocked by inserting a needle between the Achilles tendon and the superior border of the lateral malleolus and directing it toward the little toe. Infiltration is carried out as the needles are advanced toward bone.

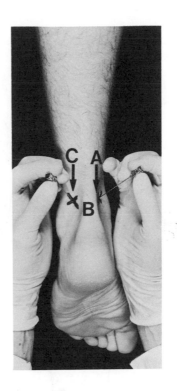

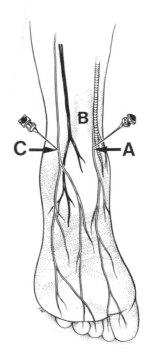

Figure 10-14. Ankle block—posterior: Anatomic drawing showing relationships and distribution of the tibial nerve **A**, Achilles tendon **B**, and sural nerve **C**.

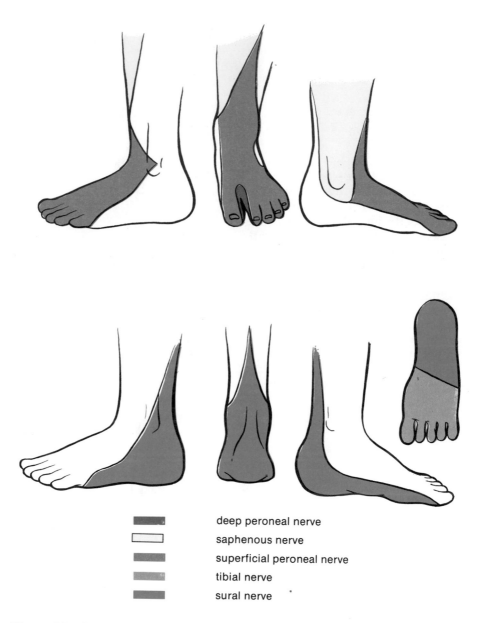

Figure 10-15. Ankle block: Cutaneous distribution of anesthesia produced by ankle block.

120

Complications

There are no complications specific to blockade of nerves supplying the foot and ankle. It may be difficult to differentiate postoperative dysesthesias secondary to needle trauma to nerves from those due to pathology or the surgical procedure. ■

11

Miscellaneous Nerve Blocks

INTRAVENOUS REGIONAL ANESTHESIA: UPPER EXTREMITY BLOCKADE

This block is in very common use for any surgical procedure performed on the arm at or below the elbow in which a tourniquet is to be utilized. The technique is so easy and the success rate so high that this block is one of the most widely utilized by both surgeons and anesthesiologists.

Most Preferred Technique

Two individual pneumatic arm tourniquets are placed as proximally as possible on the upper arm of the extremity to be blocked and connected to two separately controllable pressurized gas sources set to a pressure of at least 100 mm Hg above the patient's systolic pressure. The tourniquets should be checked prior to use to be sure they hold pressure and do not leak. A small gauge indwelling intravenous catheter is placed in the hand of the extremity to be blocked. The lumen of the catheter is then occluded with either a plastic obturator or a stopcock and the catheter is then taped in placed with minimal care since it will be removed shortly. The arm is then exsanguinated by wrapping an Esmarch bandage tightly around the fingers, wrist, and then progressively up the arm until the tourniquet is reached (Fig. 11-1). The distal tourniquet is inflated and then a few seconds later the proximal tourniquet is also inflated. The radial pulse is palpated to ensure that

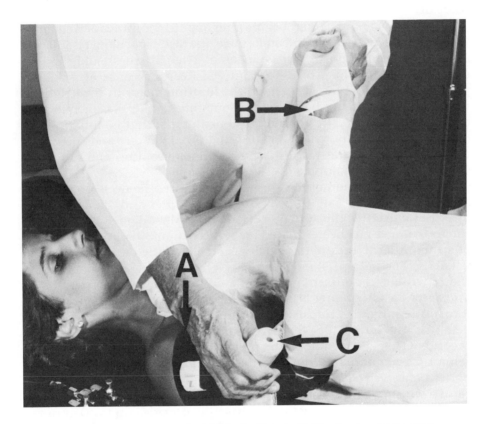

Figure 11-1. Intravenous regional block: Two individual pneumatic arm tourniquets or one double tourniquet **(A)** are placed as proximal as possible on the extremity to be blocked and connected to controllable pressurized gas sources. A small-gauge indwelling intravenous catheter **(B)** is placed in the hand of the extremity to be blocked. The arm is exsanguinated by wrapping an Esmarch bandage **(C)** tightly around the fingers, wrist, and then progressively up the arm. After inflation of the tourniquets, the Esmarch bandage is removed and 40 ml of local anesthetic are injected. Pressure is applied to the venipuncture site as the intravenous catheter is removed and pressure is continued until the arm is prepped for surgery.

arterial occlusion is complete. The distal tourniquet is then deflated and the Esmarch bandage removed. The occluding device is removed from the intravenous catheter and 40 ml of local anesthetic are injected. While pressure is applied to the venipuncture site the intravenous catheter is removed and pressure is continued until the arm is to be prepped for surgery. Satisfactory anesthesia is attained in 10 minutes. Motor blockade is often incomplete and if this is a requirement for surgery, then pancuronium 1 mg can be added to the local anesthetic solution.

Tourniquet pain usually begins after about 10 minutes of ischemia. When the patient becomes uncomfortable, the distal tourniquet is inflated and the proximal tourniquet is deflated. The patient should then be quite comfortable for up to 45 minutes. Recrudescense of ischemic pain is inevitable, however, and is the limiting factor in the length of time that ischemia can be tolerated. Sometimes, relief of ischemic pain can be accomplished by alternating tourniquets; that is, inflating the distal tourniquet and then deflating the proximal one and then vice-versa as the situation warrants. Intravenous sedation and narcotics can be very useful adjuncts in this situation.

Upon termination of the surgical procedure, the decision is made as to whether it is safe to deflate the tourniquet and allow the local anesthetic to enter the systemic circulation. Most data suggest that if the tourniquet has been inflated for greater than 30 minutes, the risk of systemic local anesthetic toxicity is small, so the tourniquet can be deflated. The patient should be observed closely. If symptoms occur, the tourniquet is immediately reinflated until the symptoms subside and then the tourniquet is cycled as follows: If less than 30 minutes of tourniquet time has elapsed, then the tourniquet should be cycled by deflating the tourniquet for ten seconds and then reinflating for 50 seconds. This cycling should be repeated several times. If the patient remains asymptomatic, the tourniquet can be finally deflated and the patient observed closely for the next few minutes. Normal sensation will return within a minute or two of final cuff deflation unless bupivacaine is used as the local anesthetic. Bupivacaine provides up to 10 minutes of postcuff-deflation analgesia (see Table 11-1).

Comments

The usual 40 ml volume of local anesthetic (for a 70kg adult) can be modified for particularly large or small patients. For example, a 35 kg child will receive good anesthesia with 20 ml. A helpful sign in determining the appropriate volume of local anesthetic to administer is the visible filling of the veins with injection of the drug.

Table 11-1
Use of Local Anesthetics for Intravenous Regional Anesthesia

Drug	Concentration (%)	Comment
Lidocaine	0.5	Most commonly used
Bupivacaine	0.25	Often provides up to ten minutes of anesthesia after tourniquet deflation
Prilocaine	0.5	Gives the lowest systemic blood levels; risk of methemoglobinemia has discouraged its use

Variations in Technique

Tourniquet

Most texts recommend the use of the standard double tourniquet which is designed specifically for intravenous regional anesthesia. The two individual pneumatic tourniquets are integrated into the same cuff unit such that each one is smaller (having smaller width) than an appropriately-sized tourniquet which would normally be utilized to provide complete hemostasis. Although they do usually work, they do not provide as reliable occlusion of arterial flow as do the standard-sized tourniquets which are recommended by these authors. This is most noticeably true when dealing with a patient with a particularly large diameter extremity. If a double tourniquet is used, then one should be especially careful to feel for an arterial pulse in the extremity after tourniquet inflation to ensure that arterial occlusion has been achieved.

Tourniquet Location

Placement of the tourniquet below the elbow, or below the knee for that matter, does not seem to provide as reliable anesthesia as when the tourniquet is placed above the elbow or knee as previously described. This is most likely due to the interosseous arterial architecture which is protected from tourniquet-induced occlusion by the surrounding bones of either the forearm or the lower leg. For this reason, this technique is not particularly recommended.

Intravenous Catheter Placement

Placement of the catheter in the dorsum of the hand is associated with a higher success rate than with placement more proximally. A lower success rate occurs with placement in the antecubital veins. This is probably due to the effect of the venous values in preventing retrograde flow of the local anesthetic to the distal extremity. Therefore, the more distally the catheter can be placed, the better the resultant block.

Occasionally the need arises to deal with a surgical situation in which it is known that the tourniquet will be deflated after a time and then reinflated, with surgery lasting a significant length of time after the second inflation. Under these circumstances, anesthesia can be restored if the intravenous catheter is not removed before the surgical prep, but rather, is isolated from the sterile field and connected to intravenous extension tubing that extends out of the surgical field. Prior to reinflation of the tourniquet, exsanguination can be accomplished by the surgeon utilizing a sterile Esmarch wrap and the catheter reinjected with one-half the dose of the local anesthetic originally injected (20 ml) which, in conjunction with the local anesthetic which remains bound in the tissues, will restore satisfactory anesthesia.

Exsanguination

In the event of a fracture of the extremity preventing the use of an Esmarch bandage, exsanguination can be accomplished satisfactorily by elevating the extremity above the heart for 5 minutes and then inflating the tourniquets as previously described.

One of the complaints of surgeons who operate under intravenous regional anesthesia is the lack of a dry surgical field. To ameliorate this problem, the "double wrap" technique has been advocated. This involves the same procedure as described under preferred technique except that, after exsanguination and before injection of the drug, a Penrose drain is applied to the forearm for procedures on the wrist and hand, forming a venous tourniquet which is left in place until one-half of the local anesthetic is injected. It is then removed and the remainder of the drug is administered. The rest of the block is performed as usual except that after the arm is prepped and draped and the proximal tourniquet has been inflated, the surgeon reexsanguinates the extremity utilizing a sterile Esmarch wrap. The distal tourniquet is inflated and the proximal tourniquet is then deflated. The authors of the original description claim an almost completely dry field and a 100% success rate with this technique.

INTRAVENOUS REGIONAL ANESTHESIA: LOWER EXTREMITY BLOCKADE

Little information is available pertaining to the success rate of intravenous regional anesthesia of the lower extremity. The general impression is that it is not as reliable. The reason for this is that most people are reluctant to inject an equivalent dose of local anesthetic into a leg because, should the tourniquet inadvertently deflate, a potentially lethal dose of local anesthetic could enter the circulation. The volume of the leg is approximately four times that of the arm, and would therefore require 160 ml of local anesthetic. In practice, most anesthesiologists inject 100–120 ml of a more dilute local anesthetic (for example, 0.25% lidocaine) to keep the total dose within a reasonable range. Tourniquet inflation pressures should be at least 200 mm Hg above the patient's systolic blood pressure to provide complete arterial occlusion with the tourniquet applied above the knee.

Mechanism of Action

There have been several studies which have tried to determine whether the site of action of intravenous regional anesthesia is at the major nerve trunks or at the peripheral nerves. The results are inconclusive and suggest that both sites are involved.

Complications

The only thing that can go wrong with this block is that it either does not work, which is unlikely, or that the tourniquet malfunctions and the patient receives an intravenous bolus of local anesthetic causing systemic toxicity. The amount of local anesthetic that enters the circulation upon tourniquet deflation is inversely related to the length of time that the tourniquet has been inflated. Therefore, the peak arterial level of lidocaine with immediate deflation is well above the seizure threshold of 12–15 μg/ml. During tourniquet inflation, there is a constant loss of local anesthetic from the venous circulation as tissue binding occurs and some drug leaks into the systemic circulation, thereby decreasing the dose suddenly released into the circulation on tourniquet deflation. After 45 minutes of tourniquet time, the arterial level produced is 2 μg/ml which should not cause any symptoms. These levels are subject to individual variation, as is attested to by the rare reports of convulsions in patients with tourniquet deflation after

45 minutes of tourniquet time. Close observation of the patient is essential. The tourniquet should remain on the patient during this observation period so that it may be reinflated at the first sign of trouble.

In discussing the pharmacodynamics of local anesthetic drugs in intravenous regional block, we are most concerned with systemic arterial levels. This is because the arterial concentration of local anesthetic is what the brain, the organ that is most susceptible to local anestetic toxicity, will be exposed to. After an intravenous bolus injection of local anesthetic, the venous levels are several times higher than the arterial levels because the lung clears a large portion of the drug on the first pass. The result is that upon tourniquet deflation after 45 minutes of intravenous regional anesthesia the venous concentration of lidocaine is 6 µg/ml while the arterial concentration is only 2 µg/ml.

Drugs themselves may produce complications. Methemoglobinemia occurs with the use of prilocaine, but recent studies would suggest that this is a safe drug when used in doses not exceeding 5 mg/kg. 2-Chloroprocaine has been implicated in the production of venous thrombosis.

FIELD BLOCK: LOCAL INFILTRATION

Anatomy

A number of minor surgical and percutaneous procedures can be performed if the terminal branches of peripheral sensory nerves are blocked. When one knows the nerve supply to the area in which work is to be done, the nerves proximal to the area can be blocked, i.e., for laceration repair, mole removal, etc. For localized lesions, one may also consider the technique of geometrically surrounding the area of operation with local anesthetic drugs placed into the intradermal and subcutaneous areas. Lastly, for some laceration repair work, infiltration of the cleaned edges of the wound will suffice.

Landmarks

The location of the pathology or the desired area of cutaneous anesthesia will dictate the site for local anesthetic infiltration. It is crucial in blocks of this kind to use epinephrine-containing local anesthetic solutions with great care because of the possibility of inducing vasoconstriction with subsequent ischemic damage to skin areas distal to the site of local anesthetic injection.

Technique

Dilute local anesthetic solutions are usually all that are necessary to provide adequate cutaneous anesthesia. If a volume in excess of 20 ml of local anesthetic is to be injected, then epinephrine 1:200,000 should be added except when digits, the nose, or the penis are to be anesthetized. A systematic approach to infiltrating intradermal areas should allow pain-free placement of needles for subcutaneous injection of local anesthetic that will result in optimal analgesia. Needles appropriate for the extent and depth of local anesthetic placement are inserted through skin wheals with injections of the drugs being made as the needle is advanced in the subcutaneous tissue. Injection should be made into the subcutaneous tissue so that the skin is slightly elevated by the local anesthetic solution. As long as the needle is in constant motion, aspiration to rule out intravascular injection is unnecessary.

INJECTION OF FRACTURE HEMATOMAS

Prompt anesthesia of a closed fracture, such as a Colles' fracture, allows relatively pain-free closed reduction and casting. This is readily accomplished by the placement of a 22-gauge needle into the fracture hematoma which is indicated by the free aspiration of blood. Ten ml of 1% lidocaine without epinephrine is injected slowly and yields good analgesia in about 5 minutes. Scrupulous aseptic technique must be adhered to since a hematoma is an excellent medium for bacterial growth. ■

Section IV

Pain Blocks

12

Sympathetic Blocks

Interruption of the sympathetic nervous system is useful for the treatment of a variety of conditions. It affords pain relief and cure in cases of reflex sympathetic dystrophy. Other names and variations of this condition are causalgia, posttraumatic syndrome, shoulder hand syndrome, and Sudeck's atrophy. Cardiac pain can be relieved by blockade of the thoracic sympathetic chain with stellate ganglion block. Cancer pain from the abdominal viscera (especially pancreatic cancer), as well as the pain of acute pancreatitis, can be relieved by celiac plexus block. Renal colic can be relieved by lumbar sympathetic block. Increased cutaneous blood flow caused by sympathetic blockade can be useful in reduction of localized edema of an extremity. Sympathetic block may also be of transient benefit in the relief of vasospastic disorders including Raynaud's disease, frostbite, or other acute vascular problems.

Anatomy

The sympathetic nervous system is supplied by preganglionic fibers from T1 to L2. After leaving the spinal cord, they travel in two paravertebral sympathetic chains that extend from the head to the pelvis. These chains give off efferent sympathetic fibers that travel to the

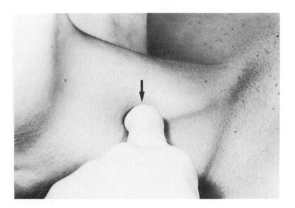

Figure 12-1. Sympathetic block—cervicothoracic (stellate): Surface anatomy of the neck with the palpating finger resting on the anterior tubercle of the transverse process of C6 (arrow) at the level of the cricothyroid notch.

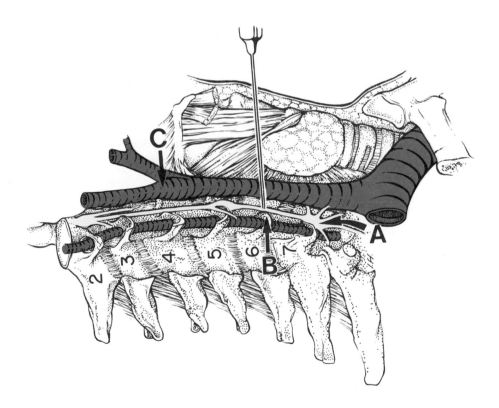

Figure 12-2. Sympathetic block—cervicothoracic (stellate): Anatomic drawing showing relationship of stellate ganglion and cervicothoracic sympathetic chain **A** to the carotid tubercle **B** and the carotid artery **C**.

extremities and to the prevertebral areas of the abdomen forming the celiac and other plexuses. Pain fibers from the abdomen, thorax, and probably the extremities as well, traverse the sympathetic chains on their way to enter the cord via the dorsal roots.

CERVICOTHORACIC BLOCK (STELLATE)

This block provides sympathetic blockade to the head, upper extremity, and organs of the chest.

Anatomy

In the cervical region, the sympathetic chain lies on the prevertebral fascia on the anterior transverse processes of the cervical vertebrae.

Landmarks

The patient is placed in the supine position with a pillow under the shoulders and the head allowed to fall into moderate extension. The patient's cricoid cartilage is then palpated. The index finger is slid down the side of the cricoid to the transverse process of C6, simultaneously retracting the carotid sheath laterally. The palpating finger then explores for the prominent tubercle of the C6 transverse process (Chassaignac's tubercle) (Fig. 12-1).

Technique

Once this important landmark has been located, the palpating finger then slides to its lateral aspect, allowing a 23-gauge needle to be inserted medial to the tubercle on the transverse process (Fig. 12-2). Once the needle encounters bone it is withdrawn 1 mm, and if aspiration has been negative, a test dose of 0.5 ml of 1% lidocaine is injected to rule out injection into the vertebral artery. If after 5 seconds there is no evidence of CNS toxicity, a volume of 5 ml is then injected, aspirating after each ml.

If at any time the patient complains of pain to the shoulder or arm, the needle has slipped posteriorly off the transverse process and is probably touching branches of the brachial plexus. If this occurs, the needle should be repositioned. A successful block of the cervical sympathetic chain is evidenced by Horner's syndrome on the injected side (miosis of the pupil, ptosis of the eyelid, anhydrosis of the side of the face, and stuffiness of the ipsilateral nares). Complete sympathetic blockade of the upper extremity requires diffusion of the local anesthetic down the sympathetic chain to the level of the second thoracic vertebra. Therefore, a Horner's syndrome may occur with no changes in skin temperature in the arm. In this instance, the block should be repeated with larger volumes.

Complications

The sympathetic chain lies in close proximity to major vascular and neurogenic structures in the neck. Block of the sympathetic chain, therefore, may produce undesirable and unexpected complications due to penetration, or run-off, of local anesthetics onto these structures.

The most serious complication of stellate ganglion block is pneumothorax. The incidence of penetration of the pleura increases exponentially when block is performed at the C7 rather than C6 level. The anterior paratracheal approach at C6 is relatively free of this complication. With pneumothorax in excess of 25%, closed pleural drainage is required. Lesser degrees of pneumothorax rarely require treatment, although patients should be warned against air travel and expulsive coughing since low atmospheric pressures increase expansion of the pneumothorax and expulsive coughing increases intrapulmonary pressure and loss of air into the pleura from small alveolar perforations.

An uncomfortable and often distressing sequela of stellate block is temporary paralysis of the ipsilateral recurrent laryngeal nerve. This produces dysphagia and a sense of fullness in the throat. The incidence of this complication (it may approach 60%) mitigates against the use of high concentrations of long-acting local anesthetics or the use of epinephrine for stellate block, since prolonged vocal cord paralysis can be extremely uncomfortable and may be associated with aspiration. If recurrent laryngeal nerve paralysis occurs, the patient should be instructed not to eat or drink until it resolves.

Phrenic nerve palsy occasionally occurs with interruption of the cervical sympathetic chain, particularly when motor blocking concentrations of local anesthetics are used. The hemidiaphragmatic paralysis is discomforting and may produce dyspnea. No treatment other than reassurance of the patient is required.

Another serious complication, that of subarachnoid block, can occur if a nerve root sleeve is entered. The extent of resultant motor or sensory paralysis depends upon the volume and concentration of the drug injected. Treatment should be expectant and dictated by the extent of block.

The vertebral artery lies in close proximity to the cervical chain as it courses through the foramen between the anterior and posterior tubercles of the transverse processes of the cervical vertebrae. Accidental injection of as little as 0.5 ml of local anesthetic into the vertebral artery will initiate seizure activity.

When large volumes in excess of 3–5 ml of local anesthetic are used for stellate block, cardioaccelerator fibers on the injected side may be blocked at the T2–4 level. In the patient with partial heart block, this may result in complete heart block. The possibility of bradyarrhythmias precludes performance of bilateral stellate block.

LUMBAR SYMPATHETIC BLOCK

This block is useful to provide sympathectomy of the lower extremity. It has no true surgical application but rather is used in the treatment of pain syndromes and vasospastic disorders or localized edema.

Anatomy

In the abdomen, the sympathetic chains lie anterolateral to the lumbar vertebrae. Since the lowest preganglionic output to the lower extremity is L2, block at that level will interrupt all postganglionic sympathetic outflow to the extremity.

Landmarks

The patient is placed in the prone position with a pillow under the abdomen or in the lateral decubitus position with the affected side uppermost. A line is drawn down the middle of the back joining the lumbar spines from L1–L5. A second line is drawn parallel to this first line at a distance of 10 cm from the midline. Where this second line intersects the lowest palpable rib is the point of insertion of the needle (Fig. 12-3).

Technique

A 6-inch, 20-gauge needle is inserted through a skin wheal at the above reference point perpendicular to the plane of the back. The needle hub is then dropped 30° laterally in the coronal plane and the needle is

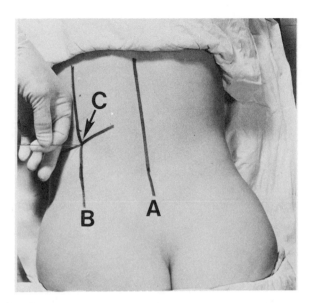

Figure 12-3. Sympathetic block—lumbar: With the patient in the prone position, a line **A** is drawn connecting the lower thoracic and all of the lumbar vertebral spines. Another line **B** is drawn parallel to line **A** 10 cm from the midline. Where line **B** intersects the lowest palpable rib is the point of the entry **C** of the needle. A 6-inch needle is introduced 30° medial from the perpendicular aiming to contact the upper border of L2 at its anterolateral aspect at a depth of approximately 5 inches. The needle is then walked off the vertebral body to advance an additional 1 cm, where 6–8 ml of local anesthetic are injected.

then advanced toward the upper third of the L2 vertebral body (Fig. 12-4). Upon contacting the body, the needle is walked off anteriorly and advanced 1 cm past the body. After aspiration in two planes, a test dose of 6 ml of short-acting local anesthetic is injected. The needle is allowed to remain in place until sympathetic blockade is demonstrated by ipsilateral increase in skin temperature. Sensory examination is then performed along the back to rule out inadvertent somatic nerve root blockade indicating incorrect needle placement. If the temperature of the extremity increases by 3°C within 3–5 minutes, 6 ml of a long-acting drug are injected.

Complications

In performance of lumbar sympathetic block, initial placement of the needle tip too superficially to the body of the vertebra may result in

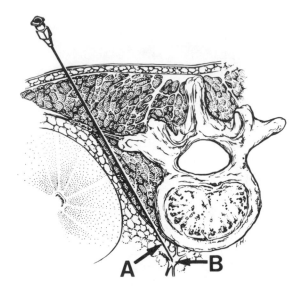

Figure 12-4. Sympathetic block—lumbar: Anatomic drawing showing the relationship of the needle **A** to the sympathetic chain **B** at the L2 level.

walking the needle into an intervertebral foramen. This may result in a subarachnoid block. If the needle tip is in the sheath of the lumbar plexus, all of the lumbar roots may be blocked.

At the level of the second lumbar vertebra, the ureters lie lateral to the vertebral body. As they descend, they assume a relationship somewhat more anterolateral to the vertebral bodies of L3 and L4 and are in close proximity to the sympathetic chain. There they are subject to injury from a sympathetic block at lower lumbar levels.

Perforation of the kidney with the 10 cm lateral approach to the sympathetic chain occasionally occurs but is of little significance. A brief period of hematuria may result but permanent damage is rare in the absence of the use of neurolytic agents.

CELIAC PLEXUS BLOCK

This block provides anesthesia of all of the abdominal viscera except for those in the pelvis and is useful for surgical anesthesia in conjunction with intercostal blocks for procedures involving the abdomen. In pain therapy it is very useful in the treatment of abdominal pain caused by pancreatitis or cancer of the viscera. Although most authors advocate bilateral needle placement, a satisfactory block will usually be obtained with unilateral block on the side most affected.

Anatomy

In the abdomen, at the level of L1, the celiac ganglia lie anterior to the vertebra and anterolateral to the aorta in a fascial compartment accessible to paravertebral needle insertion.

Landmarks

The patient is placed in the prone position with a pillow under the abdomen. The landmarks are the same as for lumbar sympathetic block. A line is drawn on the skin overlying the spinous processes from T12 to L3 and a parallel line of the same length is drawn 10 cm from the midline on the side to be blocked. The lowest (11th or 12th) rib is palpated and the intersection of the rib with the more lateral line is marked.

Technique

A skin wheal is placed just caudad to this point, and a 6-inch, 20-gauge needle is inserted through the skin wheal into the subcutaneous tissue. The needle is initially introduced perpendicular to all planes of the skin and then the needle is aimed 30° medially with the bevel down. The needle is also directed 45° in a cephalad direction so that the needle point is aimed at the anterolateral aspect of the body of the L1 vertebra (Fig. 12-5). The needle is then advanced until the vertebral body is encountered. This usually occurs at 4–5 inches in depth. If bone is encountered more superficially, the needle point may be resting on the transverse process and not the vertebral body. Once the vertebral body is encountered, the needle tip is rotated so that the bevel is toward the vertebra and is walked off anteriorly and advanced 1–2 cm beyond the vertebral body (Fig. 12-6). If the needle is properly placed, aortic pulsations will be noted.

Aspiration is performed in two planes before injecting the local anesthetic. A test dose is then injected and, after sufficient time has elapsed to rule out a subarachnoid or intravascular injection, 10 ml of short-acting local anesthetic is injected. When injecting, there should

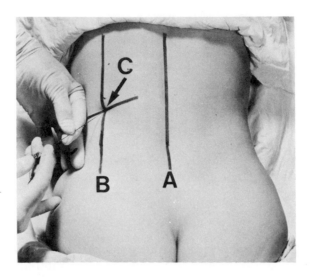

Figure 12-5. Sympathetic block—celiac plexus: With the patient in the prone position, a line **A** is drawn overlying the spinous processes of the lower thoracic and the lumbar vertebrae. A parallel line **B** is drawn 10 cm from the midline. Where this second line intersects the lowest palpable rib **C** is the point of needle entry. A 6-inch 20-gauge needle is introduced 30° medial from the perpendicular and 45° cephalad aiming at the anterolateral surface of the body of L1. When bone is contacted at approximately 5 inches, the needle is walked off the vertebral body an additional 2 cm. If the needle is properly placed, aortic pulsations will be noted in it while the breath is held. After negative aspiration, 6–8 ml of local anesthetic are injected.

be little or no resistance. Any resistance upon injection or difficulty in moving the needle in and out a few ml indicates that the tip is probably in the periosteum or the intervertebral disc rather than in the prevertebral space. After evidence of successful block (good pain relief with no evidence of somatic blockade), 10 ml of long-acting drug is injected. The needle is then withdrawn and the patient returned to the supine position. It is important to monitor the blood pressure following celiac ganglion block, as hypotension is encountered in as many as 50% of patients undergoing the procedure.

Complications

The major complication of celiac plexus block is subarachnoid block due to improper needle placement. Radiographic control during needle insertion will prevent this complication until skill in performance of

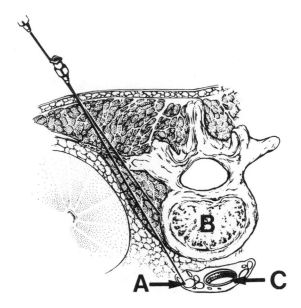

Figure 12-6. Sympathetic block—celiac plexus: Anatomic drawing showing relationship of celiac ganglia **A** to the L1 vertebral body **B** and the aorta **C**.

the block is acquired. At such time, the image intensifier is useful but not mandatory.

Too large a volume of local anesthetic may compress the aorta in its fascial compartment with the ganglia, but this complication is rare in the absence of massive tumor encroachment or chronic inflammation. Penetration of the wall of the aorta by the needle tip is indicated by gross pulsations of the needle hub and resistance to injection of the local anesthetic. With proper needle placement there should be no obstruction to flow of the injected local anesthetic. ■

13

Special Procedures

FACET BLOCK

Blockade of the nerves innervating the lumbar facet joints may provide relief from low back pain. This is usually done under X-ray control utilizing either radiofrequency or cryogenic neurolysis. Indications for the block are: pain radiating to the buttocks or sacroiliac area often made worse by hyperextension of the lumbar spine, X-ray evidence of facet arthritis, and previous response to diagnostic blocks performed utilizing local anesthetics.

Anatomy

The facet joint is innervated by the two nerves of Luschka which arise from the dorsal division of the lumbar nerves immediately above and below the joint. For example, the L4-5 facet is supplied by the posterior primary divisions of L4 and L5 spinal nerves.

Landmarks

The patient is placed in the prone position with a pillow under the iliac crests to flatten the lumbar spine. Using X-ray localization, the

142

appropriate vertebral body level is identified. The needle insertion point will lie over the base of the transverse process immediately below the facet joint to be blocked. This is usually 2.5-inches lateral to and at the inferior margin of the spinous process just cephalad to the transverse process previously identified. For example, to block the L4-5 facet, the needle insertion point is about 2.5-inches lateral to the L4 spinous process (Fig. 13-1).

Technique

A 3.5-inch needle is inserted at the point described above, perpendicular to the skin in all planes. If local anesthetic is to be injected for diagnostic purposes, then a 3.5-inch, 22-gauge spinal needle is usually best. The needle is inserted until contact is made with the base of the spinous process. The needle is then directed slightly medially and walked into the posterior aspect of the joint. Recreation of the patient's pain with needle placement or upon electrical stimulation confirms correct needle position. Two ml of local anesthetic is used for diagnostic purposes at each level. Cryoprobe needles may be left in situ, and if pain relief occurs, neurolysis is carried out (Fig. 13-2).

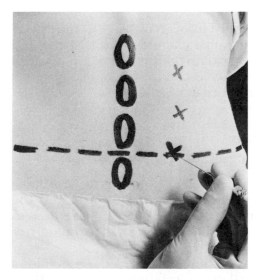

Figure 13-1. Facet block—landmarks: The needle entry point for L4-5 facet blockade is 2.5 inches lateral and at the level of the inferior margin of the L4 spinous process (dotted line). The needle is directed slightly medial and cephalad into the facet joint under radiographic control. Subsequent levels are blocked in a similar fashion.

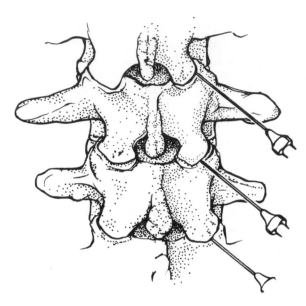

Figure 13-2. Facet block: Anatomic drawing showing relationship of needles to the facet joints.

Complications

Entry of the needle into a root sleeve at the intervertebral foramen with production of subarachnoid block is the major complication of facet block. Close proximity of the needle tip to the posterior primary ramus of the spinal nerves may result in weakness of the back muscles if the block is performed at several levels.

EPIDURAL STEROIDS

A common procedure for the management of pain due to nerve root irritation as is commonly seen in disc disease is the use of epidural steroid injections. The depot steroids employed decrease the edema and inflammation of traumatized and entrapped spinal nerve roots, thereby decreasing pain and increasing mobility.

Best results are obtained when epidural steroids are used for: *acute* intervertebral disc herniation with true radiculopathy with sensory, motor or reflex changes and electromyographic or contrast myelography evidence of a bulging disc. Results under these conditions compare favorably with disc surgery. Chronic low back pain or postlaminectomy pain responds less well.

Technique

For a herniated lumbar disc, the patient is placed in the lateral decubitus position with the affected side recumbent. The level of nerve root entrapment is identified and marked (L5-S1 for an S1 radiculopathy, L4-5 for L5, L3-4 for L4, since it is the developing, rather than the emerging, root that is entrapped). After sterile preparation an epidural block is performed with a 17- or 18-gauge Tuohy Huber needle by loss of resistance technique. When the epidural space is identified, a mixture of 3–5 ml of 1% lidocaine mixed with 50 mg of triamcinolone diacetate (2 ml) is slowly introduced. Paresthesias along the course of the entrapped root are often encountered and are modified by decreasing the speed of injection. The needle is then withdrawn and the patient maintained in the lateral position for 15 minutes. Patients should be advised that as the local anesthetic is absorbed from the injection site, pain may return for a period of up to 24 hours before the steroid becomes effective.

The patient should be evaluated at 2 weeks following block for any change in neurological findings. If there is total lack of sustained improvement or any increase in neurological findings, immediate further diagnostic studies are required. If the patient has improved in both signs and symptoms, no further block is performed, but the patient is reevaluated in 2 more weeks. If the patient is improved but has reached a plateau, the block may be repeated on the return visit. Follow-up is continued in this fashion, but rarely are more than three blocks required. Caution is advised regarding injection of depot steroids in a greater dosage or at more frequent intervals because of the hazards of adrenal suppression, fluid retention, and psychic disturbances.

SUPRASCAPULAR BLOCK

Suprascapular block interrupts the sensory pathways from the shoulder capsule and joint and provides relief of shoulder pain. This allows rapid institution and progression of physical therapy in treatment of shoulder disability.

Anatomy

The suprascapular nerve derives from the superior trunk of the brachial plexus and contains root fibers from the 5th and 6th cervical segments. It runs caudad and lateral to the upper border of the scapula at which point it passes through the suprascapular notch and runs laterally beneath the suprascapularis muscle to the lateral border of the spine of the scapula. It then penetrates the infraspinous fossa and divides into its terminal branches. The nerve is a mixed nerve, the motor branches supplying the supra- and infraspinatus muscles. The sensory fibers supply the acromioclavicular articulation and the tendinous cuff of the shoulder joint. These fibers end in terminal filaments supplying the posterosuperior portion of the shoulder joint. The nerve is most accessible to blockade at the suprascapular notch, where it passes under the transverse scapular ligament.

Landmarks

The suprascapular notch is most readily located by identification of the tip of the acromion and the medial border of the scapula at the level of the scapular spine. These points are marked and a line is drawn between them that corresponds to the spine of the scapula. This line is then bisected and a point marked 1 cm cephalad to the spine. This is the point of entry of the needle to approach the suprascapular notch (Fig. 13-3).

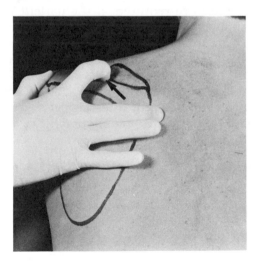

Figure 13-3. Suprascapular block: The midpoint of the superior border of the spine of the scapula is marked (arrow). A 22-gauge spinal needle is inserted perpendicular to all planes of the skin to contact the medial inferior border of the suprascapular notch at approximately 5 cm. A marker is advanced on the needle to 1.5 cm from the skin surface. The needle is then withdrawn to the subcutaneous tissue and redirected 10° laterally and cephalad and advanced to the depth of the marker into the suprascapular notch where 5 ml of local anesthetic are injected. On occasion, it may be necessary to walk the suprascapular blade to identify the notch.

Technique

A skin wheal is raised 1 cm above the midpoint of the scapular spine. A 3-inch, 22 gauge spinal needle with stylet in place is introduced perpendicular to all planes of the skin until bone is contacted at the medial border of the suprascapular notch at a depth of approximately 3 cm. A marker is then set at 1.5 cm from the skin. The needle is then withdrawn to the subcutaneous tissue, redirected 15° lateral and 15° cephalad and introduced towards the suprascapular notch to the depth of the marker (Fig. 13-4).

Because of anatomic variations, the needle may drop into the notch on initial insertion. This may be detected by an increase in resistance as the needle penetrates the suprascapular ligament in excess of 3 cm depth. It may also be necessary to walk the needle laterally or medially or more cephalad along the scapula superior to the spine if the notch is not found. When the notch is located and entered by the needle, 5 ml of local anesthetic of a sensory concentration are introduced after negative aspiration. This block is effective in interrupting all afferent impulses from the shoulder joint, bursae, and tendinous cuff.

Complications

The most common complication is block of the motor branches to the supraspinatus muscle when too high a concentration of local anes-

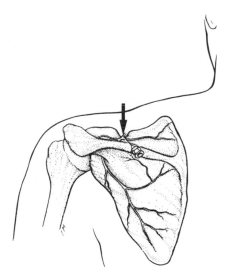

Figure 13-4. Suprascapular block: Anatomic drawing showing location of suprascapular notch (arrow) and distribution of the suprascapular nerve.

thetic is used. This results in inability to initiate abduction of the arm at the shoulder joint. Insertion of the needle through the notch to a depth greater than 1.5 cm may find the needle point in contact with the brachial plexus on the first rib, resulting in a brachial block. Close attention to the depth of needle insertion and avoidance of insertion in a caudad direction will prevent penetration of the pleura.

OCCIPITAL NERVE BLOCK

Occipital nerve blocks provide anesthesia of the skin of the occiput and relieve the headache associated with tension or spasm of the cervical muscles and pain of C2 nerve root irritation.

Anatomy

Cervical nerves leave the spinal cord horizontally at the level of the corresponding vertebral body and above the intervertebral disc. As the first cervical nerve leaves the spinal canal between the atlas and the occiput, it lies in a groove of the first cervical transverse process beneath the vertebral artery. The posterior primary division of the first cervical nerve then joins with the second to form the greater occipital nerve. This conjoined nerve runs dorsally under a triangle formed by the inferior oblique, superior oblique, and rectus capitis posterior major muscles.

The sensory branches then pierce the semispinalis capitis and the trapezius muscles at the base of the skull and accompany the occipital artery to supply the skin and underlying tissues over the posterior portion of the scalp as far as the vertex. The branches enter the superficial fascia at the level of the superior nuchal line of the occipital bone 2.5 cm from the external occipital protuberance.

The lesser occipital nerve arises from the posterior primary division of the second and third cervical nerves and may also have a contribution from the fourth nerve. The main trunk divides into medial (cutaneous) and lateral (muscular) branches. The medial branch passes backward and, piercing the sternocleidomastoid muscle, supplies the skin of the posterior surface of the pinna of the ear and the adjacent portion of the scalp.

Landmarks

Block of the greater occipital nerve is facilitated with the patient in the seated position. The patient is requested to flex the head with the chin on the chest, bringing into prominence the bulk of the upper fibers of the trapezius muscle where they attach to the superior nuchal line. Points just lateral to the trapezius insertion 1.0 cm below the occiput and 2.5 cm from the external occipital protuberance are palpated and marked for the greater occipital nerves (Fig. 13-5).

The lesser occipital nerve is located just lateral to the posterior border of the insertion of the sternocleidomastoid muscle into the skull. Figure 13-6 demonstrates the relationship of the greater and lesser occipital nerves to the surrounding structures.

Technique

For block of the greater occipital nerve, a 1.5-inch, 23-gauge needle with syringe attached is inserted through the skin, subcutaneous tissue, and muscle from the above-marked points in a cephalad direction to contact bone just caudad to the superior nuchal line. The needle is then withdrawn slightly from the bone and, after negative aspiration, 3 ml of local anesthetic are deposited at each site.

Lesser occipital nerve block is performed by inserting the 1.5-inch, 23-gauge needle just lateral to the mastoid process and in a cephalad

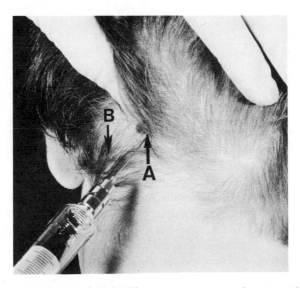

Figure 13-5. Occipital nerve block: The greater occipital nerve is located by marking the point **A** at the posterior nuchal line just lateral to the erector muscles of the neck. The lesser occipital nerve **B** is located at the posterior nuchal line just posterior to the mastoid process. The needle should be inserted in a cephalad direction and the anesthetic solution injected in a transverse fanwise manner from these points.

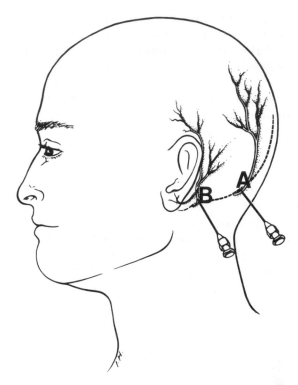

Figure 13-6. Occipital nerve block: Anatomic drawing showing relationships and distribution of the greater **(A)** and lesser **(B)** occipital nerves. (Reproduced from Carron H: Control of pain in the head and neck. Otolaryngol Clin North Am 14(3), August 1981.With permission.)

direction to contact bone caudad to the superior nuchal line. The needle is then withdrawn slightly, and after negative aspiration, 3 ml of local anesthetic are injected.

An alternate approach to the lesser occipital nerve can be used if the greater is to be blocked as well. After injection of the greater occipital nerve, the needle is withdrawn to the subcutaneous tissue and redirected to contact bone at the base of the skull just posterior to the mastoid process. Withdrawing the needle slightly, 3 ml of local anesthetic are injected.

Complications

Complications of occipital nerve block are related primarily to accidental intravascular injection. With the volume of local anesthetic used, intravenous injection is of little consequence. The same volume injected into the occipital artery, however, may travel retrograde and produce a transient convulsion. If too long a needle is used and it is directed medially, it is theoretically possible for the needle to enter the foramen magnum with consequent cisternal block or trauma to the brain stem.

LATERAL FEMORAL CUTANEOUS NERVE BLOCK

Lateral femoral cutaneous nerve block provides analgesia of the lateral thigh and can be used to provide cutaneous anesthesia of that area or for the treatment of meralgia paresthetica which sometimes follows lower abdominal surgery.

Anatomy

The lateral femoral cutaneous nerve is derived from the L2 and L3 roots of the lumbar plexus. It has a long course through the pelvis, being lateral to the psoas muscle and immediately inferior to the ilioinguinal nerve. It runs in an oblique and ventral direction along the medial side of the iliacus muscle. Although it occasionally will run through the inguinal ligament, it usually passes deep to the ligament at the distance of approximately 1–2 fingerbreadths medial to the anterior superior iliac spine (ASIS). From this location, it courses to the lateral thigh at the origin of the sartorius muscle, where it is covered by the fascia lata. It divides into the anterior and posterior branches to provide sensation to the anterolateral aspect of the thigh.

Landmarks

The patient is placed in the supine position and the ASIS is identified, as is the inguinal ligament. A mark is placed on the skin that is approximately 2 cm medial and 2 cm caudad to the ASIS (Fig. 13-7). Figure 13-8 shows the relationship of the nerve to the anterior superior iliac spine.

Technique

A 1-inch, 23-gauge needle, or a 1.5-inch, 22-gauge needle, is inserted perpendicular to all planes to the skin at the mark previously made. One will likely feel the give of the needle as it passes through the fascia that overlies the lateral femoral cutaneous nerve. Once this has been felt, 10–15 ml of local anesthetic solution is injected with a slight in-and-out and lateral to medial movement of the needle. An additional injection may be made to block the nerve as it exits the pelvis. For this, the needle is aimed laterally to contact the iliac bone. Then it is withdrawn and guided in a slightly more medial direction to a depth that is

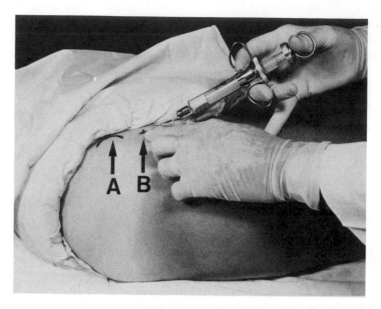

Figure 13-7. Lateral femoral cutaneous nerve block—landmarks: **A** indicates the anterior superior iliac spine. Needle entry point **B** is 2 cm medial and 2 cm caudad to point **A**.

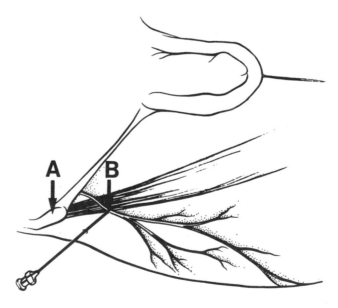

Figure 13-8. Lateral femoral cutaneous nerve block: Anatomic drawing showing relationship of the anterior superior iliac spine **A** to the nerve **B**.

152

approximately 2.5 cm deeper than where bone was previously touched. An additional 10 ml of local anesthetic solution is injected after aspiration of the needle is negative for blood.

Complications

Repeated needling and block of the lateral femoral cutaneous nerve may result in prolonged dysesthesia or hypesthesia of the anterolateral aspect of the thigh.

TRIGGER POINTS

There are localized areas in either muscles or ligaments or both that may be painful to palpation. Although the exact etiology of trigger points is not always obvious, direct musculoskeletal trauma and chronic muscle stress from tension, abnormal posture, and fatigue are common causes. Trigger points can occur in any muscle, ligament, or fascial area, but are most common in the posterior cervical paraspinal muscles, the low back muscles, the upper anterior chest muscles, and surgical scars.

Landmarks

Trigger points are usually easily identified because of the severe pain elicited with palpation. In addition to the pain produced, one may appreciate that the involved muscle feels tight or bandlike.

Technique

The patient is placed in a comfortable position that allows ready access to the trigger point. A 1-inch, 23-gauge needle, or a 1.5-inch, 22-gauge needle, depending upon the perceived depth of the structure in which the trigger point lies, is inserted through the skin that overlies the trigger point. A skin wheal may be placed beforehand. The needle is advanced until the patient's pain is reproduced or at least until the painful intramuscular area has been located. Then the needle is aspirated. If negative for blood, 2–4 ml of local anesthetic solution with or without 1–2 ml of a depot steroid preparation are injected.

INTRAVENOUS SYMPATHECTOMY

Intravenous guanethidine (15 mg in 23 ml of normal saline with 500 units of heparin) has been found to produce a sympathetic blockade of the upper extremity which persists for 3 days. The technique is similar to that described for intravenous regional anesthesia except that only a single tourniquet is applied to the extremity and it remains inflated for only 15 minutes after the injection of the guanethidine.

Sympathetic blockade of the lower extremity is accomplished with 20 mg in 48 ml of normal saline with 1,000 units of heparin. Unfortunately, this promising technique for the treatment of Raynaud's phenomenon and the sympathetic dystrophies is not currently available as guanethidine is not approved for intravenous use in the United States. Instead, reserpine 1.25 mg can be used to provide a sympathetic block of shorter duration for the upper extremity. Side effects such as diarrhea and fatigue can occur with this drug.

EPIDURAL NARCOTICS

The early enthusiasm for the profound analgesia provided by narcotics injected into the epidural space has been dampened by the side effects of itching, urinary retention, nausea, and sedation, but, most particularly by delayed, severe respiratory depression which may occur many hours after a single dose of narcotic, particularly morphine. There have been several reports of respiratory arrest. The current use of these techniques should be restricted to situations where the patient can be monitored closely as long as the risk of respiratory depression exists.

Doses of 5–10 mg of preservative-free morphine in 10 ml of normal saline are injected through an epidural catheter after a test dose of 50 mg of lidocaine containing 25 μg of epinephrine fails to produce tachycardia or subarachnoid block. Pain relief without orthostatic hypotension can be expected to last 12–20 hours depending on the dose.

Implantable continuous infusion devices may offer relief of intractable pain from advanced malignancy in selected patients. It is hoped that exploitation of new knowledge of opiate receptors and the development of new drugs will result in safer and more widespread use of this promising technique for the control of pain. ■

14

Neurolytic Blocks

The use of neurolytic blocks should be reserved for permanent interruption of autonomic fibers. Only in the treatment of cancer pain
in the terminal patient is the interruption of somatic pathways
justified.

It should be cautioned that the loss of sensation produced by a
local anesthetic bathing nerve roots or peripheral nerves is not the
same as that produced by neurolytic agents. Local anesthetics interrupt
impulse transmission at the site of action of the drug. Peripheral neurolysis produces retrograde nerve degeneration that may extend through
the ventrolateral tracts to the thalamus. The long-term peripheral man-
ifestation is then one of dysesthesia or anesthesia dolorosa, which is
often more discomforting to the patient than the original pain.

Neurolytic agents in common use are alcohol, used in concentrations ranging from absolute (100%) to 25% in water or normal saline,
and phenol 6–7% in water or oil contrast medium and 10–20% in
glycerine. Neurolytic agents in low concentrations are anesthetic, but
in higher concentrations cause denaturation of proteins. Nerve
destruction is directly related to the concentration of the drug. Sensi-
tivity of individual fibers to varying concentrations lacks confirmation.

The affinity of vascular tissue for phenol is greater than that of its affinity for nervous tissue. Conduction defects from more dilute solutions may therefore be related to destruction of small vessels supplying nervous tissue rather than interruption of the nerves themselves.

TREATMENT OF SPASTICITY

Neurolytic agents have been used for the control of spasticity. Dilute solutions of aqueous phenol (2–3%) or ethyl alcohol (45%) have been utilized. These solutions interrupt the gamma loop reflex and thereby reduce muscular spasm.

The most common technique seeks for the motor end plates with sheathed needles and a stimulator and injection is then carried out with small volumes (0.1–0.2 ml) of alcohol or phenol until adequate relief of spasticity is noted. Another technique injects large quantities of 45% alcohol (20–40 ml per muscle group) in a "shotgun" fashion across the belly of a spastic muscle until relaxation occurs (Fig. 14-1). Unfortunately, the duration of relief of spasticity is short, varying from 2 months to a year. Neurolytic blocks, however, are useful when used

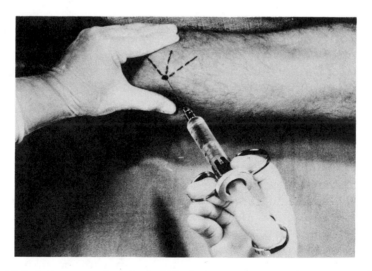

Figure 14-1. Intramuscular alcohol block: For treatment of spasticity, the muscle is maintained in a state of spasm or clonus by forced extension. A 22-gauge spinal needle is introduced into the spastic muscle and 45% ethyl alcohol (U.S.P.) is injected in a fanwise direction across the belly of the muscle. Injection should be continued until sudden relaxation is noted (20–30 ml per muscle group).

in conjunction with muscle stretching and physical therapy. Complications, including deep venous thrombosis, painful neuritis, and muscular weakness are common.

PERIPHERAL NERVE BLOCKS

Intercostal blocks with neurolytic agents for pain relief in metastatic disease involving the ribs can be justified by the fact that the duration of effect frequently exceeds life expectancy. No more than two intercostal nerves below T6 should be blocked, since abdominal musculature will be denervated, resulting in abdominal wall weakness. Injection must be carried out intraneurally, however, since neurolytic agents have low diffusibility.

EPIDURAL INJECTION

In rare instances of malignancy involving a single spinal nerve root, the use of 10% phenol in glycerine in the epidural space will provide pain relief with minimal motor dysfunction. With the patient in the lateral decubitus position and the affected side recumbent, 2 ml of the phenol solution are slowly introduced at the level of root emergence from the spinal canal. The patient is maintained in the lateral recumbent position for 30 minutes before being permitted to ambulate. The glycerine permits localization of the phenol to the affected root due to its high specific gravity. While the literature is sparse on the results of epidural phenol injection, our experience has shown that pain relief persists for 2–4 months following injection. *The use of epidural alcohol is not recommended,* since its spread cannot be controlled.

INTRATHECAL INJECTION

Absolute alcohol and phenol (5–10%) in glycerine or contrast medium have been used for the treatment of pain due to malignancy and the relief of spasticity of spinal cord injury or multiple sclerosis. Subarachnoid neurolytic block is not recommended for pain of benign origin.

Since alcohol is hypobaric to spinal fluid, the patient must be positioned so that the affected nerve root is uppermost (Fig. 14-2). The subarachnoid space is entered with a 25-gauge needle at the level of nerve root emergence and 0.5–1 ml of 1% lidocaine is injected to determine if pain relief ensues. The patient should be retained in this position until anesthesia from the lidocaine is dissipated. Absolute alcohol

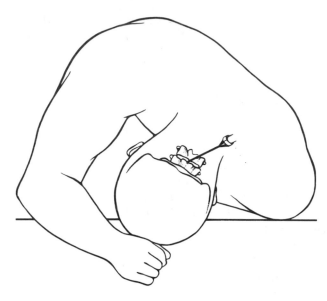

Figure 14-2. Subarachnoid alcohol neurolysis: The patient is placed in a semiprone position with the affected area uppermost. Subarachnoid puncture is performed at the selected interspace through which the root to be blocked exits. Preferably a 25- or 26-gauge, short bevel spinal needle should be used through an introducer. When spinal fluid is obtained, increments of 0.1 ml of absolute alcohol are introduced into the subarachnoid space. The needle stylet is replaced following each injection and the patient checked for dermatomal sensory loss. Additional increments of 0.1 ml may be added, to a maximum of 0.5 ml. When satisfactory pain relief is obtained, the needle is removed and the patient retained in the same position for an additional 45 minutes. (Reproduced from Carron H: Control of pain in the head and neck. Otolaryngol Clin North Am 14(3), August 1981. With permission.)

is then injected in 0.1 ml increments at 3–5 minute intervals until pain is relieved. Under no circumstances should more than 0.5 ml of alcohol be used.

If the patient is properly positioned, the alcohol will float on the spinal fluid and contact the affected nerve root and root entry zone as it enters the dorsal horn (Fig. 14-3). The patient should be maintained in the original position for 30 min following injection.

Phenol in glycerine is hyperbaric in spinal fluid. Hence, the patient must be so positioned that the affected nerve root is more dependent. To perform a dorsal root block, the patient is placed in the lateral position with the affected side dependent. A 22-gauge needle is placed in the intrathecal space at the level of the affected nerve root and the

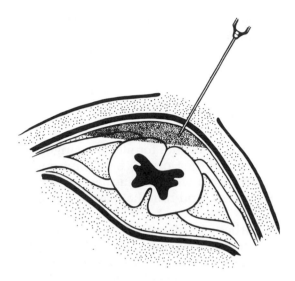

Figure 14-3. Subarachnoid alcohol neurolysis: Anatomic drawing showing the floating of the hypobaric alcohol on the spinal fluid to involve the dorsal sensory root and the dorsal root entry zone of the spinal cord. (Reproduced from Carron H: Control of pain in the head and neck. Otolaryngol Clin North Am 14(3), August 1981. With permission.)

patient is rotated 60°–70° supine. Increments of 0.1–0.2 ml of 10% phenol in glycerine are injected at 3–5 minute intervals until pain relief is obtained. One-half ml of phenol in glycerine is the maximum dose to be used for sensory root blockade.

When intrathecal phenol in glycerine is to be used to decrease spasticity due to spinal cord injury, a 22-gauge spinal needle is introduced at least two segments below the patient's sensory level. The patient is then tilted 80° toward the prone position with the affected side dependent and with the head of the table slightly elevated. Two ml of 10–20% phenol in glycerine is injected. The patient is maintained in the above position for 30 minutes. This will produce blockade primarily of the unilateral ventral nerve root. For bilateral block, the patient is placed in the full prone position. Intrathecal phenol for relief of spasticity provides more prolonged effect when higher concentrations (15–20%) of phenol in glycerine are used. Our experience has been that spasticity is relieved for 4–24 months and repeat blocks are equally effective.

Results of subarachnoid block for pain relief are extremely variable, with good results ranging from 25–65%. Unfortunately, in the patient with metastatic disease, relief of the most predominant pain frequently unmasks a secondary pain. One then finds himself in the position of chasing the pain through repeated neurolytic blocks, often leaving the patient with increasing muscle weakness as well as bladder and bowel dysfunction.

SYMPATHETIC BLOCKS

The use of neurolytic agents for stellate ganglion block is *not* recommended. Patients find the Horner's syndrome and nasal congestion unacceptable. Potential runoff to the cardiac acceleration fibers, recurrent and phrenic nerves, and brachial plexus present additional hazards.

Lumbar sympathetic block with 50% alcohol or phenol (6–7%) in water or contrast medium has had wide application despite continued reports of serious complications. Most misadventures have occurred when the sympathetic chain was blocked below L2.

While it is generally recommended that lumbar sympathetic block be performed under radiographic control, there is little evidence that the incidence of complications is less than that by the blind technique. It is essential that the block be first performed with a single needle at the L2 level with a small volume (6–8 ml) of short-acting local anesthetic. The onset of a 3°C rise in temperature of the foot on the blocked side within 3 minutes indicates proper needle placement. Failure to obtain the 3°C temperature rise necessitates replacement of the needle and repetition of the local anesthetic block. When proper positioning of the needle has been ascertained, the local anesthetic can be followed with 6–8 ml of 6% phenol in water. The needle should then be cleared with saline or local anesthetic to avoid leaving a phenol tract.

Neurolytic celiac plexus block can be performed with 8 ml of neurolytic agent on a single side if the needle is placed within the fascial compartment containing the aorta and celiac ganglia. As with lumbar sympathetic block, the use of a local anesthetic prior to use of a neurolytic agent is essential. The unmedicated patient with abdominal pain of malignancy can readily determine relief from the local anesthetic. The use of local anesthesia prior to alcohol (50%) or phenol (6%) in water permits the operator to determine whether the needle is in the intervertebral foramen, viscera, or blood vessel.

TRANSSACRAL NEUROLYSIS

The detrusor muscles of the bladder are controlled by the sacral roots S2-4. Selective denervation of a dominant root decreases urgency, frequency and bladder spasm in the contracted or inflamed urinary bladder. Individual sacral roots are blocked in a predetermined sequence with 2 ml of 0.25% bupivacaine and the patient observed for 24 hours following block of each sacral root until the dominant nerve is identified. When a single root block produces improvement in symptoms, that root is then blocked with 1–1.5 ml of 6% phenol in water. Improvement varies from 4–18 months, at which time the procedure can be repeated. In the incontinent patient post abdominoperineal resection with perineal tumor recurrence, bilateral S4 blocks with 1.5 ml of 6% phenol in water at each site will provide several months of pain relief.

COMPLICATIONS

Complications of lumbar sympathetic block include subarachnoid injection and damage to viscera (see Complications of Lumbar Sympathetic Block, in Chapter 12). As the ureter descends into the pelvis, it moves from its lateral position in the renal fossa to a position at L3 anterolateral to the body of the vertebra in close relationship to the sympathetic chain. Injection of neurolytic agents at L3 or L4 has a high liability for ureteral damage with necrosis and formation of a neuroma.

The most significant complication of transsacral nerve block, particularly at the S1 and S2 levels, is penetration of the end of the dural sac. Injection of neurolytic agents into the sac will produce permanent anesthesia of the perineum and urinary and fecal incontinence. Vascularity of the sacral space requires special care that intravascular injection does not occur.

Complications of celiac plexus block are outlined on page 122. In addition, because of its high affinity for vascular tissue, phenol may erode the aorta. It is probably preferable to use 50% alcohol for performance of this neurolytic block. Unilateral neurolytic block with small volumes of drug causes little hypotension, other side effects being minimal as well. ∎

Section V

Enhancing Regional Techniques

15

Preparation

POSITIVE APPROACH TO THE PATIENT

Most anesthesiologists would prefer regional over general anesthesia for a surgical procedure performed on themselves. They are the most knowledgeable as to the relative risks and advantages of both techniques. Most patients, on the other hand, request general anesthesia. They are less knowledgeable and should be educated by the medical establishment. A common statement made by patients who refuse spinal anesthesia, for example, is that they are afraid because of stories they have heard about patients being paralyzed from the procedure. In the 10-year period from 1948–1958, 582,190 spinal anesthetics were reported with no permanent motor paralysis observed. The incidence of *any* neurological complications (most of which are transient) associated with spinal or epidural blockade is estimated to be about 1:11,000. The *mortality* due to complications of general anesthesia is also estimated to be about 1:11,000. These figures, while crude approximations, justify the clinical impression that properly conducted regional anesthesia may cause less physiologic trespass upon the patient than does general anesthesia.

It is with this attitude that the fears of the patient should be dispelled by the truth presented in a supportive manner. Patients should be assured that they will receive any desired sedation during the procedure to make the experience in the operating room a pleasant one.

PREMEDICATION AND INTRAVENOUS SUPPLEMENTATION

There are no hard and fast rules in regard to premedication and intravenous supplementation with sedatives and narcotics. The desired end point is a calm, cooperative patient. This is best achieved by an informative and supportive preoperative visit, and then appropriate premedication tailored to the needs of the patient. A particularly anxious patient may benefit from a relatively large oral dose of one of the benzodiazepines. Upon arrival in the operating suite, further doses of intravenous benzodiazepines should be given until the patient is calm, but not so sedated that response and assistance cannot be elicited during the performance of the block.

After placement of the block, intravenous narcotics may be given for any discomfort that may arise from the performance of the block or any discomfort that may arise during the surgical procedure, such as that which occurs from lying in one position for a prolonged period. Appropriate supplementation will avoid the often encountered problem of the over-anxious patient interpreting any stimulus as pain. Readily available narcotics such as fentanyl and benzodiazepines will greatly increase the success rate for regional anesthesia.

OPERATING ROOM PREPARATION: TIMING AND EQUIPMENT

Regional anesthesia takes time. Other than spinal blockade, most regional techniques require at least 20 minutes before surgical levels of anesthesia are obtained. Some techniques take even longer. The milieu in the operating room is seldom conducive to waiting. Therefore the patient, when possible, should be brought to an induction area at least a half hour before the start of the surgery. Intravenous access should be established and vital signs taken. The block may then be performed and allowed to set up in a controlled, unhurried atmosphere. Under these conditions, assessing the block and then performing any additional supplemental blocks as necessary after an appropriate waiting period (usually 10–15 minutes) will greatly improve the overall success rate.

An induction area should contain all necessary safety equipment, including oxygen and positive pressure delivery systems (bag and mask), airways, suction, facilities for measuring blood pressure (and ECG when possible), and drugs for the treatment of complications: ephedrine for hypotension, sodium pentothal or diazepam for therapy of CNS local anesthetic toxicity, and succinylcholine to provide paralysis and allow establishment of an endotracheal airway during local anesthetic-induced convulsions.

pH ADJUSTMENT OF LOCAL ANESTHETICS

Commercial preparations of local anesthetics containing epinephrine have relatively low pH's. When sodium bicarbonate is added to the solutions to increase the pH to about 7, significantly faster onset and more intense blocks are obtained with little change in duration. Earlier work by Bromage using carbonated lidocaine and more recently by Galindo using sodium bicarbonate added to commercial anesthetic solutions substantiate these findings. The mechanism hastening the onset and intensity of local anesthetics is thought to occur by increasing the proportion of local anesthetic present in the unionized (inactive but highly diffusable) form, which causes greater membrane penetration. In addition, the rapid diffusion of carbon dioxide into the nerve tissue may cause an ion trapping effect by providing a relatively acidic medium inside the nerve. When the unionized anesthetic solution reaches the nerve, it is therefore converted to the ionic (anesthetically active, poorly diffusable) form which is trapped inside the nerve. Other factors such as very high pCO_2 may also contribute to inhibition of nerve conduction.

To prepare pH adjusted local anesthetic solutions of lidocaine or mepivacaine, 1 mEq of sodium bicarbonate is added to each 10 ml of anesthetic solution. This will yield a pH of approximately 7. Greater quantities of sodium bicarbonate will cause the anesthetic to precipitate as the pH increases above 7. Bupivacaine is pH adjusted by adding 0.1 mEq of sodium bicarbonate to each 10 ml of anesthetic solution immediately before injecting. The bupivacaine will precipitate slowly once pH adjusted, and so should be used immediately.

In summary, this relatively new technique appears to offer shorter set up times, denser blockade, and greater success rates than when low pH, commercially prepared solutions are used. Caution should be exercised in regard to dosage and toxicity until further studies are available to indicate whether significant differences exist between these and standard commercially prepared solutions. ■

16

Needles

CHOICE OF NEEDLES

Short-beveled needles are preferred because they are not as sharp as the standard, long-beveled ones and are therefore less apt to injure nerves. Also, the tip of a short-beveled needle is closer to the end hole (Fig. 16-1), so the injection of local anesthetic will more likely be in the same tissue plane as the tip. This is particularly important if a paresthesia caused by touching the needle tip to the nerve is used to localize the nerve prior to the local anesthetic injection. The duller, short-beveled needles also provide a better feel as the needle traverses the different tissue planes.

A 1.5-inch, 22-gauge, short-beveled needle is usually preferred for most superficial blocks as it provides sufficient rigidity and ease of injection. The Becton-Dickenson B bevel needle is the most commonly used. For deeper blocks, longer needles are required. Twenty-two-gauge needles longer than the standard 3.5-inch spinal needle are too flimsy to allow precise placement. Twenty-gauge needles are then usually preferred.

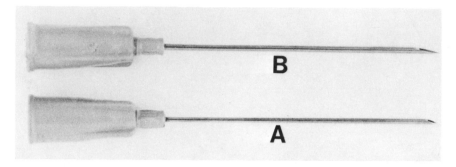

Figure 16-1. Needles for nerve block: Short-beveled needles **(A)** are preferred over standard, long-beveled needles **(B)** because they are duller and hence less likely to injure a nerve. They also provide a better "feel" and the opening (eye) of the needle is closer to the tip, enhancing the accuracy of the block. (Needles manufactured by Monoject, St. Louis, MO).

USE OF NEEDLES

Immobile Needle Technique

The use of a length of intravenous connecting tubing connected to the needle allows an assistant to aspirate and inject local anesthetic solutions without any significant movement of the needle (Fig. 16-2). One of the physician's hands is, therefore, freed up so that one hand may be used for palpation or retraction while the other grasps the needle. This technique is generally used when needle movement is likely and needle tip position needs to be precisely maintained.

Walking Off of Bone

When walking off of bone into the appropriate location, the bevel should be directed so that the needle tip slides off rather than digs into the periosteum. If walking off bone (and periosteum) causes significant patient discomfort, then 1–2 ml of local anesthetic should be injected prior to proceeding further. Usually, the faster the needle is walked, the less discomfort the patient will experience.

NERVE LOCALIZATION

Seeking Paresthesias

Probably the most common technique used to localize a nerve is the eliciting of a paresthesia by touching the needle to the nerve. This provides a painful dyesthesia or paresthesia for the patient. Adequate

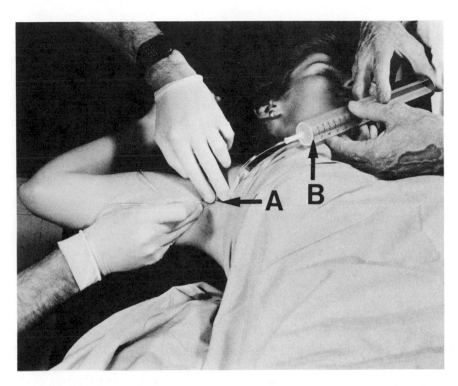

Figure 16-2. Immobile needle technique: The needle **(A)** is connected to the syringe **(B)** by intravenous connecting tubing. An assistant can then aspirate and inject at the direction of the physician, thus preventing unwanted needle movement.

sedation and instruction will decrease the patient's withdrawal from the pain as the needle reaches its target. The patient is instructed to say, "Now," when he first feels the paresthesia and to describe its radiation. If the paresthesia is in the correct location corresponding to the nerve distribution that is sought, the needle is held immobile, and after negative aspiration, 1 ml of local anesthetic is injected slowly and the patient is asked whether this produces further paresthesias. If it does, then the injection is presumed to be at least partially into the nerve and the needle is withdrawn 1 mm and another 1 ml of solution is injected. This procedure is repeated until no paresthesia is obtained upon injection. An intraneural injection will produce increased resistance to local anesthetic injection. When the needle tip is determined to be next to, but not in, the nerve, a test dose of local anesthetic (3–5 ml) is injected to rule out an intravenous injection. After waiting 30 seconds for symptoms of systemic toxicity, the remainder of the local anesthetic is injected slowly with frequent repeated aspiration, usually after every 5 ml.

The best technique for eliciting a paresthesia is to thoroughly learn the anatomy of the area and be able to feel the needle tip's passage through the various tissue planes. The course of the nerves should be determined and any accompanying structures such as arteries palpated to help localize the nerve. The needle should be inserted slowly such that the nerve will not be harpooned by the sharp point of the needle. The most effective method for searching for a paresthesia is fanning with gentle, rapid, small incremental changes in needle direction in the plane perpendicular to the course of the nerve.

A common pitfall in searching for a paresthesia occurs when a pain-sensitive structure other than the desired nerve is touched. For example, when, periosteum is contacted it causes pain, which may be referred distally in a manner suggestive of a paresthesia. The most helpful means of differentiating these is by knowing the sensory distribution of the nerve to be blocked and comparing it to the radiation of the pain reported by the patient. Also, referred pain usually does not radiate past the next most distal joint of an extremity as does a true paresthesia. For example, in performing an axillary block of the brachial plexus, the paresthesia obtained should extend below the elbow to be considered valid. In children or very anxious adult patients uncomfortable paresthesias may be undesirable and other means of nerve localization, such as motor nerve stimulation, may be preferred. ■

17

Nerve Stimulators

MOTOR NERVE STIMULATION

These techniques rely upon attaching a nerve stimulator to the needle to depolarize the motor fibers of the nerve. This causes contraction of the muscles in the motor distribution of the nerve. The advantage of this technique is that patient discomfort is minimal and cooperation is not required. With higher voltages, the stimulator can also produce motor nerve stimulation while the needle tip is several centimeters from the nerve. The resultant muscle contractions will increase in intensity as the needle homes in on the nerve. Disadvantages are that more equipment is required and that, when standard needles are used, the placement of the needle tip may not be as close to the nerve as when a paresthesia is obtained.

A nerve stimulator such as that used to monitor neuromuscular blockade, with one of the two leads fitted with an alligator clip, is utilized (Fig. 17-1). One of the two leads is attached to an ECG pad placed away from the area to be blocked. The other lead, with the alligator clip, is attached at the hub of the needle whereupon the needle is inserted through the skin. The voltage control, usually graduated from 0–10, is turned up until the muscles underlying the electrocardiogram pad or

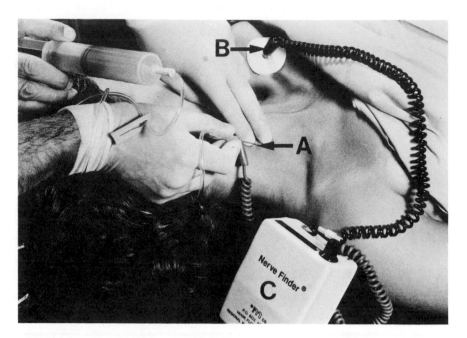

Figure 17-1. Nerve stimulator: A nerve stimulator allows location of nerves by motor stimulation. **A** indicates the needle with alligator clip from the stimulator attached at the hub, **B** the other stimulator lead attached to an ECG electrode placed on the opposite side of the body from the extremity to be blocked, and **C** the nerve stimulator with voltage control knob. As the needle is advanced, the extremity is observed for motor activity consistent with the nerve stimulated.

needle can be seen or felt to contract during stimulation (the stimulator should be set to stimulate one time per second). The needle is advanced toward the nerve until muscle contractions in the appropriate motor distribution occur and the voltage is then turned down to just above threshold to obtain motor stimulation. The needle thus homes in on the nerve, as is demonstrated by increased intensity of muscle contractions as the needle tip approaches the nerve. The optimum needle position is determined by the greatest motor stimulation with the minimum voltage setting, whereupon 2 ml of local anesthetic are injected. The motor contractions will decrease following injection. If the contractions do not recur after 30 seconds, the needle tip can be presumed to be in the correct position close to the nerve and further injection may take place.

Refinement of this technique is possible using needles which are insulated except at the very tip. This allows more precise localization

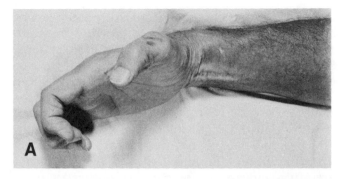

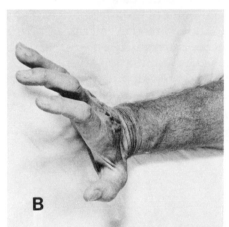

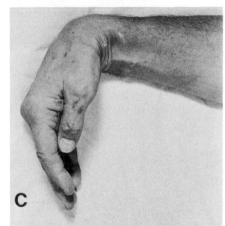

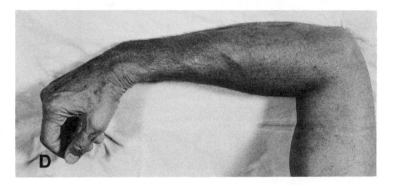

Figure 17-2. Nerve stimulator: Upper extremity movements seen with motor stimulation of the nerves arising from the brachial plexus. **(A)** Stimulation of the median nerve produces flexion of the fingers and wrist. **(B)** Stimulation of the radial nerve produces extension of the wrist and elbow. **(C)** Stimulation of the ulnar nerve produces flexion of the metacarpophalangeal joints and the wrist. **(D)** Stimulation of the musculocutaneous nerve produces flexion of the elbow.

173

during electrical stimulation. In addition, stimulators are now available which provide direct readings of current flowing through the needle. This allows better localization since muscle contractions with lower current thresholds (less than 1.0 mamp) imply that the needle must be very close to the nerve. Higher thresholds imply that the needle is farther away.

The motor innervation of the muscle groups to be stimulated should be learned prior to initiating the block. For example, stimulation of the nerves of the brachial plexus produces the movements shown in Figure 17-2. (A-D) Stimulation of a muscle directly by a needle may cause an entire extremity to move and should not be confused with correct needle placement near a nerve. The exact movements produced by the nerve should be sought. As a general rule, the motor movements seen with direct stimulation of a muscle will not occur beyond the next most distal joint in contrast to contractions caused by stimulation of a nerve.

Other techniques of nerve localization rely upon knowledge of the anatomy of the local region and are discussed in conjunction with specific nerve blocks. ■

Section VI

Complications

18

Systemic Complications

The major complications of regional anesthesia are related to the systemic effects of high blood levels of the local anesthetics or to neurologic damage. Other physiologic derangements related to high spinal blockade may result in morbidity and mortality if inadequately treated.

DRUG ABSORPTION AND SYSTEMIC EFFECTS

High blood levels of local anesthetics can occur with accidental intravenous or arterial injection or, in a slower time course, absorption from perineural sites. Absorption produces blood levels directly related to the blood flow at the injection site and the amount of drug injected. From a given dose of drug, blood levels are highest with intercostal blocks, lowest with spinal and axillary blocks, and intermediate with epidural and caudal blocks. For example, the general range of blood levels to be expected for each 100 mg of lidocaine injected will vary from 0.5 μg/ml to 1.5 μg/ml depending on the site injected. A quick rule of thumb is that for each 100 mg of lidocaine given epidurally, a 1 μg/ml blood concentration results. If the same dose is given for an intercostal block, the blood level is 50% higher (1.5 μg/ml), and if given for subarachnoid block, it is 50% less or 0.5 μg/ml.

Blood levels of local anesthetics are important in that they are predictive of systemic effects. The systemic toxicity of these drugs occurs when certain critical levels are achieved in brain and heart. As an example, the effect of lidocaine blood concentration will be considered. The effect on the brain is dose-related and paradoxical. At low blood levels such as 1–5 μg/ml, lidocaine produces an anticonvulsant effect. At these blood levels, lidocaine also has effective antiarrhythmic, antitussive and mild sedative effects which reduce anesthetic requirements. With these levels, the symptoms commonly reported by the patient include ringing in the ears and circumoral numbness. The EEG at this level is that of light sleep.

At higher blood concentrations, i.e., 12–15 μg/ml for lidocaine and 4–6 μg/ml for bupivacaine, seizures will occur. The prodrome before seizures includes slow speech, jerky movements, tremors and hallucinations. The EEG will have spike wave activity with slow waves. The seizures originate in the amygdala and hippocampus and spread centrally. The treatment of the seizures consists primarily of preventing tissue hypoxia. This is achieved by establishing adequate ventilation using 100% oxygen. Suppression of the seizures can then be produced by raising the seizure threshold with either diazepam or thiopental. Succinylcholine can be used to facilitate adequate ventilation. The choice among these drugs will depend on the patient's status and whether cardiac depression is present.

At very high blood levels, 20–25 μg/ml for lidocaine, toxic effects on the cardiorespiratory system occur in man. Respirations become shallow and rapid. Blood gases will reflect respiratory acidosis. As the upper concentration range is achieved, apnea occurs. Hypotension develops and is followed by cardiovascular collapse. Therapy in such patients should be directed toward maintenance of respiration and circulation (CPR) once collapse occurs.

Although lidocaine was used as the model for the effects of various blood levels of local anesthetics on the brain and heart, similar effects are produced by other local anesthetics. In general, lidocaine and mepivacaine are essentially equivalent in activity and toxicity. Etidocaine and bupivacaine are 2–4 times as potent as lidocaine in producing local anesthesia, and seizures are produced at blood levels roughly one-fourth that of lidocaine. The managment of toxic symptoms secondary to elevated local anesthetic concentrations is identical regardless of the local anesthetic involved.

Evidence in animal studies suggests that the ratio between seizure and cardiorespiratory depressant effects is relatively constant for the local anesthetics. Recent studies have demonstrated that all commonly used local anesthetics produce a concentration-related depression of intraatrial, AV nodal, intraventricular conduction, and myocardial contractility. The more potent agents depress conduction and contractility at significantly lower concentrations than the less potent local anesthetic drugs. Reports have appeared where severe cardiac toxicity occurred due to bupivacaine shortly after the onset of seizures. Furthermore, some of these patients have been resistant to cardiac resuscitation.

HYPOTENSION

The most common complication of regional anesthesia following subarachnoid or epidural block is hypotension, the extent of which depends upon the level of sympathectomy. The higher the level of block, the greater the degree of hypotension. Total sympathectomy is usually achieved with a sensory level of T4. Compensation occurs by vasoconstriction above the level of the block, and therefore, the higher the level of sympathectomy, the fewer the compensatory areas of vasoconstriction available.

Cardiovascular changes that occur are a decrease in preload from dilatation of the major capacitance veins, a decrease in afterload from arteriolar dilatation, and a decreased heart rate and ionotropic state with total sympathectomy, causing resultant inhibition of cardioaccelerator fibers. The change in preload is of greatest importance. The overall myocardial oxygen balance with moderate levels of hypotension due to spinal anesthesia is favorable, with myocardial demand lowering more than supply. Cardiac output is maintained at normal levels despite a 20% decrease in mean arterial pressure. Therefore, overzealous treatment of moderate hypotension is to be discouraged. If the mean arterial pressure decreases beyond moderate levels (30%) or the patient becomes symptomatic from CNS or coronary hypoperfusion, then aggressive therapy should be pursued.

The most prompt treatment of sudden hypotension due to sympathectomy is elevation of the lower extremities, but not the steep Trendelenburg position. Leg elevation increases the circulating blood volume as much as 750 ml. In the Trendelenburg position, in the presence of profound hypotension the venous pressure may increase excessively, decreasing cerebral perfusion pressure and thus interfering with cerebral blood flow. The rapid infusion of 200–300 ml of balanced salt solution will usually assist in returning the systolic pressure to acceptable levels in the presence of *gradually* developing hypotension. When the pressure fall is abrupt, intravenous fluids should be supplemented with increments of a dual-acting vasopressor, such as ephedrine, in 10-mg increments. ■

19

Neurologic Complications

Despite fears of permanent neurologic sequelae of regional anesthesia, the incidence of nerve damage or paralysis is quite rare. Most neurological derangements regress with time, but may be a cause for concern in the occasional patient.

POSTDURAL PUNCTURE (SPINAL) HEADACHE

Postdural puncture headache following subarachnoid or epidural blockade is probably the most frequent and troublesome problem following regional anesthetic procedures. Low pressure (spinal) headache is due to loss of cerebrospinal fluid. Its frequency is directly related to the size of the needle used. Approximately 10 ml of CSF per hour is lost following a 22-gauge needle puncture. The fluid loss causes the brain to sag when the patient is in the upright position, producing traction on cerebral vessels. The onset of headache occurs 24–48 hours following subarachnoid puncture and is characterized by occipital and frontal headache, cervical muscle spasm, and nausea and vomiting when erect. The headache usually disappears on assuming the recumbent, prone, or supine position. Enforced recumbency in the immediate postoperative period fails to prevent spinal headache.

Low pressure headache usually resolves spontaneously in less than 2 weeks, but intractable headache may require hydration, analgesics, or epidural blood patch with 10–15 ml of autologous blood. To perform an epidural blood patch, the epidural needle should be inserted at the same level as the previous lumbar puncture. When the epidural space has been identified, 10–15 ml of the patient's blood is withdrawn from an antecubital vein under aseptic precautions and then introduced slowly through the epidural needle. The venous needle should be left in place and one to two liters of balanced salt solution infused during the ensuing 60–120 minutes. The patient should be retained in the recumbent position for approximately 1 hour following the patch. If the headache recurs during the ensuing 48 hours, the blood patch can be repeated. Complications of this procedure are notably absent and relief is usually prompt and complete with a single injection in 95% of patients.

High-pressure headache, characterized by its persistence regardless of position, may occur from meningeal irritation due to septic or aseptic meningitis.

Cranial nerve palsies occurring following subarachnoid puncture are also due to loss of cerebrospinal fluid, with consequent traction on cranial nerves. Abducens palsy (6th cranial nerve) is most common and usually resolves in a matter of weeks.

NERVE INJURY

Serious neurological lesions occur with trauma to nerve roots or the spinal cord or are secondary to injection of irritant drugs. The accidental intraneural injection of local anesthetics into nerve roots may, by a hyperosmolar effect, cause denaturation of proteins. The phenomenon has been demonstrated with 10% dextrose and 10–20% procaine in dogs.

The spinal roots are under tension from their derivation at the spinal cord to their exit at the intervertebral foramina and do not readily move out of the way as the needle is introduced into the subarachnoid space. Paresthesias during subarachnoid puncture, therefore, suggest that the needle has impinged a nerve root. Any persistent paresthesia demands that the needle be withdrawn and repositioned. A clear, free flow of spinal fluid is a requisite for injection.

Since 1980, there have been reports of several cases of transient and permanent neurological changes in patients who had received accidental intrathecal injection of large volumes of 2-chloroprocaine. Animal investigations since that time have revealed that the changes seen with 2-chloroprocaine or its vehicle are similar to those found with other local anesthetics, namely macrophage infiltration of the meninges and subpial necrosis of the spinal cord. These changes have also been found in animals that showed no neurological deficits. Explanations for this phenomenon are lacking, but have led to the suggestion that epidural injections of local anesthetics should be incremental (5 ml per injection) and that, should accidental perforation of the dura occur and a large volume be injected, CSF should be drained in an amount equivalent to the volume of injected anesthetic.

Nerve trauma occurs when nerve fibers are directly needled or when highly concentrated local anesthetic agents are injected intraneurally. In many regional anesthesia procedures it is common to seek paresthesias, but injection of local anesthetic should be discontinued promptly if the patient complains of a paresthesia during injection.

If a patient demonstrates sensory or motor alteration following a regional anesthetic procedure, it is essential that EMG studies be done promptly as part of a complete neurological examination to document the baseline neurological status of the patient. Denervation changes do not occur for 7—14 days and an EMG can assist in ruling out preexisting nerve injury. The EMG also provides a convenient method of following the course of nerve regeneration and reinnervation.

Epidural hematoma with cord compression and resultant paraplegia is the most feared complication of epidural block. It occurs most frequently in elderly patients in whom epidural pressures are greater and more prolonged following local anesthetic injection or bleeding. Progressing neurological deficit from suspected epidural hematoma is a true neurosurgical emergency requiring myelography and decompression. Among the other infrequent complications of epidural block are epidural abscess, mechanical trauma to nerve roots, backache, and neurological deficits secondary to injected drugs.

Anterior spinal artery syndrome has been attributed to the use of vasopressors in conjunction with spinal anesthetic drugs. The use of epinephrine probably should be avoided in the elderly and atherosclerotic patient, although a causal relationship has not been established. Arachnoiditis has been known to follow the use of high concentrations of local anesthetics and dextrose and the inadvertent injection of sclerosing substances into the subarachnoid space. This may result in the development of the cauda equina syndrome with disturbances in gait and bladder and bowel function accompanied by pain. ■

20

Technical Complications

Technical complications relate either to breaks in aseptic technique or to faulty or contaminated equipment.

BACKACHE

Backache is fairly common following surgical procedures regardless of the anesthetic used. It is usually related to prolonged supine position on the operating table with loss of the normal lordotic curve incident upon anesthesia and relaxants. With spinal and epidural analgesic techniques, the needle may traumatize the periosteum or facets of the vertebral bodies. On occasion, a spinal needle may enter and traumatize an intervertebral disc. Trauma to the soft tissues themselves may produce low back discomfort for variable periods.

BROKEN NEEDLES AND CATHETERS

Needles may break if contacting bone or when attempts are made to change their direction without first withdrawing to a more superficial plane. Security bead needles obviate the loss of portions of needles in deep tissue, but tend to be more fragile at the bead site. Segments of needles must be removed either magnetically or surgically since they tend to migrate.

Catheters used for continuous techniques are most vulnerable to breakage at the skin and at the needle tip where the sharp bevel may shear a catheter that is being incorrectly withdrawn through the needle. Catheters may also curl back on themselves, making their removal difficult. Small sections of broken *epidural* catheters may not require removal since they are constructed of inert materials. Broken sections of *subarachnoid* catheters should be removed surgically to prevent possible neurologic damage.

PROLONGED BLOCK

The clearance of drugs from tissue spaces is a function of blood flow and hence the duration of analgesia from a fixed drug mass will vary between individuals. The range, however, is fairly constant. The presence of competitive drugs, however, may markedly affect the duration of analgesia. Drugs competing for cholinesterase will prolong the effect of the ester group of local anesthetics. Drugs such as cimetidine or propranalol may prolong the effect of lidocaine through decreasing plasma clearance by the liver. Patients with demyelinating diseases such as diabetes mellitus, alcoholism, multiple sclerosis and amyotrophic lateral sclerosis may develop extremely dense and prolonged blocks with local anesthetics.

HEMORRHAGE

Bleeding is not uncommon when needles traumatize highly vascular areas such as the epidural space, the head and neck, genitalia, and other loose areolar tissues. Bleeding is increased in the presence of anticoagulants, in patients on high doses of salicylates, and in patients with bleeding disorders due to systemic disease.

Particularly vulnerable are those deeper areas invaded for sympathetic blockade. Retroperitoneal hemorrhage can occur following lumbar sympathetic and celiac block and large cervical hematomata may follow attempts at stellate ganglion block.

SPILLOVER

Spillover of local anesthetics onto nerves other than those being blocked is usually of minor consequence, although occasional serious problems may arise. Recurrent laryngeal and phrenic block have already been alluded to previously. Spillover during lumbar sympathetic block occurs with inexact needle placement and can involve the somatic fibers of the lumbar plexus, producing limb weakness.

A high epidural or subarachnoid block may interrupt cardioaccelerator and cervical sympathetic fibers, resulting in profound bradycardia or bilateral Horner's syndrome. Involvement of adjacent nerves is of greatest consequence when neurolytic agents are used, since partial denervation of somatic nerves can result in discomforting dysesthesias and complete interruption can interfere with function.

LOCAL EFFECTS

Local tissue trauma can result from multiple needle punctures, the introduction of contaminants, necrosis from high drug concentrations, or excessive volumes of local anesthetics containing epinephrine. Traumatized tissue is particularly susceptible to infection and abscess formation may occur. This is of major significance when the abscess occurs in the epidural space. Local anesthetics injected into infected and acidotic areas will often fail to produce satisfactory anesthesia.

SUMMARY

The hazard of any invasive procedure is inversely proportional to the time and care spent in preparation for and performance of the technique. Careful and scrupulous attention to detail in regional anesthesia will minimize complications and untoward results. Patient complaints or neurological deficits following nerve blocks should be investigated immediately and carefully documented. ■

Suggested Readings

Anatomy

Cousins MJ, Bridenbaugh PO (Eds): Neural Blockade in Clinical Anesthesia and Management of Pain. Philadelphia, JB Lippincott Co, 1980

Ellis H, Feldman S: Anatomy for Anaesthetists. London, Blackwell Scientific Publications, 1979

Eriksson E (Ed): Illustrated Handbook in Local Anaesthesia (ed 2). Philadelphia, WB Saunders Co, 1980

Greene NM: Physiology of Spinal Anesthesia (ed 2). Baltimore, Williams & Wilkins Co, 1969

Moore DC: Regional Anesthesia. Springfield, Charles C Thomas Publishers, 1975

Moore DC, Bush WH, Burnett LL: Celiac plexus block: A roentgenographic anatomic study of technique and spread of solution in patients and corpses. Anesth Analg 60:369–379, 1981

Moore DC, Bush WH, Scurlock JE: Intercostal nerve block: A roentgenographic anatomic study of technique and absorption in humans. Anesth Analg 59:815–825, 1980

Netter FH: The Ciba Collection of Medical Illustrations, vol 1, Nervous System. New York, Ciba, 1962

Pansky B: Review of Gross Anatomy. New York, MacMillan Pub Co, 1979

Pick J: The Autonomic Nervous System. Philadelphia, JB Lippincott Co, 1970

Romanes GJ (Ed): Cunningham's Textbook of Anatomy (ed 10). London, Oxford University Press, 1964

Technique

Boas RA: Sympathetic blocks in clinical practice, in International Anesthesiology Clinics. Boston, Little, Brown & Co, 1978, pp 149–182
Bonica JJ: The Management of Pain. Philadelphia, Lee & Febiger, 1953
Bonica JJ: Principles and Practice of Obstetric Analgesia and Anesthesia, vol 2. Philadelphia, FA Davis Co, 1969
Bromage PR: Epidural Analgesia. Philadelphia, WB Saunders Co, 1978
Carron H, Korbon GA: Common nerve blocks in anesthetic practice. Seminars in Anesthesia 2:30–49, 1983
Carron H, Litwiller R: Stellate ganglion block. Anesth Analg 54:567–570, 1975
Cousins MJ, Bridengaugh PO (eds): Neural Blockade in Clinical Anesthesia and Management of Pain. Philadelphia, JB Lippincott Co, 1980
Eriksson E (Ed): Illustrated Handbook in Local Anaesthesia (ed 2). Philadelphia, WB Saunders Co, 1980
Moore DC: Regional Block. Springfield, Charles C Thomas Publishers, 1973
Thompson GE: Pharmacology, physiology, and use of spinal and epidural anesthesia. Seminars in Anesthesia 2:24–29, 1983
_____: Symposium on intravenous regional anesthesia. Reg Anesth 4, Jan–Mar 1979
_____: Symposium on regional anesthesia for upper extremity surgery. Reg Anesth 5, Jan–Mar 1980

Special Procedures

Brechner T: Percutaneous cryogenic neurolysis of the articular nerve of Luschka. Reg Anesth 6:18–22, 1981
Bromage PR, Burfoot MF, Crowell DE, Truant AP: Quality of epidural blockade. III. Carbonated local anesthetic solutions. Br J Anaesth 39:197, 1967
Carron H: Control of pain in the head and neck, in Johns ME, Rice DH (Eds): Otolaryngologic Clinics of North America, vol 14, no. 3. Philadelphia, WB Saunders Co, 1981
Carron H: Relieving pain with nerve blocks. Geriatrics, 33:49–57, 1978
Carron H, Toomey TC: Epidural steroid therapy for low back pain, in Stanton-Hicks M, Boas R (Eds): Chronic Low Back Pain. New York, Raven Press, 1982
Galindo A: pH adjusted local anesthetics—clinical experience (Abstract). 8th Annual Meeting American Society Regional Anesthesia, 1983, p 25
Galindo A, Galindo A: Spinal needle for nerve blocks. Reg Anesth 5:14–21, 1980
Haas LM, Landeen FH: Improved intravenous regional anesthesia for surgery of the hand, wrist and forearm, the second wrap technique. J Hand Surg 3:194–195, 1978
Raj PP, Rosenblatt R, Montgomery SJ: Use of the nerve stimulator for peripheral blocks. Reg Anesth 5:14–21, 1980
Rosenblatt PM, Cress JC: Modified Seldinger technique for continuous interscalene brachial plexus block. Reg Anesth 6:82–84, 1981
Rosenblatt RM: The air test for regional blocks. Anesthesiology 51:95, 1979

Selander D, Edshage S, Wolff T: Paresthesiae or no paresthesiae: Nerve lesions after axillary block. Acta Anaesth Scand, 23:27–33, 1979

Sharrock NE, Bruce G: An improved technique for locating the interscalene groove. Anesthesiology 44:431–433, 1976

Simon DL, Carron H, Rowlingson JC: Treatment of bladder pain with transsacral nerve block. Anesth Analg 61:46–48, 1982

Complications

Bridenbaugh PO: Complications of regional anesthesia. ASA Annual Refresher Course Lectures, ASA, Park Ridge, 1980

Bromage PR: Complications and contraindications, in Epidural Analgesia. Philadelphia, WB Saunders Co, 1978

Covino BG, Marx GF, Finster M, Zsigmond EK: Prolonged sensory/motor deficits following inadvertent spinal anesthesia (Editorial). Anesth Analg 59:399–400, 1980

deJong RH: Local Anesthetics. Springfield, Charles C Thomas Publishers, 1977

Greene NM: Physiology of Spinal Anesthesia. Baltimore, Williams & Wilkins Co, 1981

Katz J, Aidinia SJ: Complications of spinal and epidural anesthesia. J Bone and Joint Surg 62:1219–1222, 1980

Liu P, Feldman HS, Covino BM, Giasi R, Covino BG: Acute cardiovascular toxicity of intravenous amide local anesthetics in anesthetized ventilated dogs. Anesth Anal 61:317–322, 1982

Liu P, Feldman HS, Covino BM, Giasi R, Covino BG: Acute cardiovascular toxicity of procaine, chloroprocaine and tetracaine in anesthetized ventilated dogs. Reg Anesth 7:24–29, 1982

Mazze RI, Dunbar RW: Plasma lidocaine concentrations after caudal, lumbar epidural, axillary block, and intravenous regional anesthesia. Anesthesiology 27:574–579, 1966

Moore DC: Complications of Regional Anesthesia. Springfield, Charles C Thomas Publishers, 1955

Moore DC: Etiology, identification and treatment of systemic toxic reactions (Abstract). 7th Annual Meeting American Society of Regional Anesthesia, 1982, pp 98–103

Orkin FK, Cooperman LH (Eds): Complications in Anesthesiology. Philadelphia, JB Lippincott Co., 1983

Saidman LJ, Moya F (Eds): Complications of Anesthesia. Springfield, Charles C Thomas Publishers, 1970

Swerdlow M: Complications of local anesthetic neural blockade, in Cousins MJ, Bridenbaugh PO (Eds): Neural Blockade in Clinical Anesthesia and Management of Pain. Philadelphia, JB Lippincott Co, 1980, pp 526–542

Swerdlow M: Medicolegal aspects of complications following pain relieving blocks. Pain 13:321–331, 1982

Index

A

Abdominal blocks, 82–95. *See also specific blocks*
Abdominal wall, anesthesia of, 76
Abdominal surgery, 46, 139, 151
Amputation, of forefoot, 116
Anatomy
    of brachial plexus block, 16–17, 20, 23
    of celiac plexus block, 139, 141
    of cervical plexus blocks, 10
    of cervicothoracic block, 133, 134
    of elbow block, 96–97
    of epidural block, 46–47
    of facet block, 142, 144
    of ilioinguinal, iliohypogastric, and genitofemoral blocks, 85–86, 87
    of intercostal block, 76
    of lateral femoral cutaneous nerve block, 151, 152
    of local cutaneous blocks, 128
    of lower extremity blocks, 106
    of lumbar plexus block, 27, 29
    of lumbar sympathetic block, 136, 138
    of occipital nerve block, 148
    of obturator nerve block, 82–83
    of paracervical block, 91, 92
    of penile block, 93, 94
    of pudendal nerve block, 88, 89
    of subarachnoid block, 34
    of suprascapular block, 145–146
    of sympathetic nervous system blocks, 132–133
    of transsacral block, 64, 65
    of trigeminal nerve block, 68–69, 73
    of wrist block, 100, 102

U

V